Dedicated to my father

Nelson S. Bole

ACKNOWLEDGEMENTS

The author wishes to express his appreciation to his Committee Chairman, Dr. Donald L. Avila, for his sage advice and counsel, and to the other members, Dr. Walter Busby and Dr. Richard Anderson, for their scholarship, friendship and guidance.

The author also wishes to thank the faculty of the Human Services Department at Santa Fe Community College, Gainesville, Florida, for their support of this research. Special thanks to Dr. William Korth for his support and to Maria Duncan for her creative suggestions and help throughout the development of this research. Also, thanks to the Human Services' student volunteers who were the subjects of this experiment.

Special thanks to Alec Riddle, University of South Carolina, for his cooperation in offering research information which was most helpful to the author.

Grateful mention must also be made of Dr. Paul Schauble, University of Florida Counseling Center, for his advice and aid in providing raters for this research. Thanks to David Linquist and Gabriel Rodriquez who served as the raters.

Finally, the author expresses his deepest gratitude to his father for his untiring support and encouragement.

TABLE OF CONTENTS

LIST OF TABLES

LIST OF TABLES (Continued)

Abstract of Dissertation Presented to the Graduate Council
of the University of Florida in Partial Fulfillment of the
Requirement for the Degree of Doctor of Philosophy

THE EFFECT OF THE RELAXATION RESPONSE ON THE
POSITIVE PERSONALITY CHARACTERISTICS OF
PARAPROFESSIONAL COUNSELORS

By

David Nelson Bole

March 1978

Chairman: Donald L. Avila
Major Department: Foundations of Education

This study hypothesized that there would be measurable
gains in self-actualizing values of a group of student paraprofessionals as a result of the regular practice of the
Benson Relaxation Response (RR), a meditation technique.
It was further hypothesized that such gains would be associated with increased proportions of facilitative responses
on the parts of these students, acting as counselors, in
reacting to the communications of fellow-students, acting
as clients.

The study was carried out during the winter semester of
1977 when a group of volunteers who were students in their
first term at Santa Fe Community College were randomly
assigned to two groups: 14 to an experimental group
and 8 to a control group. The experimental group practiced
RR throughout a 10 week period while the control group did
not.

viii

Both groups were pretested by use of the Shostrom Personal Orientation Inventory, which is believed to measure values that have been associated with self-actualization and positive mental health. Research cited indicates a correlation between many of the values measured by the POI and counselor effectiveness.

In measuring changes in proportion of facilitative responses the unit of analysis employed was the level of content in the counselor's response to client communication of four dichotomized dimensions as rated on the Counselor Verbal Response Scale (CVRS): (a) Affective/Cognitive; (b) Understanding/Nonunderstanding; (c) Specific/Nonspecific; and (d) Exploratory/Nonexploratory. Each member of the population made a pretest tape at the beginning of the study which was compared with a posttest tape made at the end.

Significant gains in self-actualization by the RR group vis-a-vis the NRR group were found in five of the POI scales. Significant gains were also made in the posttest scores of the RR group compared with its pretest scores. No gains in any self-actualizing values were found in the NRR group.

Significant gains by the RR group in their proportion of facilitative responses were found only in the area of understanding of the client's responses. However, in spite of the absence of significant gains, as measured by the "t" test statistic, in any of the other CVRS scales, the RR posted impressive percentage gains in the proportion of their facilitative responses on all CVRS scales. And when the facilitative response proportion of all the scales was combined, the mean group proportion showed significant gains by the RR group.

It was concluded that the Benson Relaxation Response is one method for acquiring and developing the positive personality traits which have been linked to effective counseling and resulting client growth. In terms of counselor behavior that is measured by the CVRS scale, the initial results of RR practice may be a gain in the capacity for understanding another person's verbal communication, rather than in the other areas which may depend more on specific training and experience than on stage of personality development.

CHAPTER I

INTRODUCTION

Purpose of the Study

The purpose of this study was to examine the effects of
a meditation technique upon the behavior of a group of paraprofessionals acting as counselors. The specific behavior
examined was the counselor's responses to client communications in terms of four dichotomized dimensions: (a) affective-
cognitive; (b) understanding-nonunderstanding; (c) specific-
nonspecific; and (d) exploratory-nonexploratory. (See
Appendix B.) The meditation technique used was that
developed by Benson. It was used to test meditation as a
method of developing and improving skills related to effective counseling as well as to enhancing those perceptual
attitudes and personality traits correlated with effective
counseling performance.

Background of the Study

Paraprofessionals

Community services, such as care for the physically,
emotionally and intellectually handicapped all require far

1

more trained manpower than professional schools have been producing. To meet this need programs have been established to train Human Services' personnel who, working under professional supervision, can provide such necessary services as counseling and interviewing.

The recognition and acceptance of this need for counseling services has rapidly accelerated over the last twenty years. Counseling services have become an integral part of programs aimed at the educational, vocational, and psychological well-being of the individual. As a result of this growth, both the training and use of a new body of workers have been the target of increasing research. These workers are referred to as "support personnel," "lay helpers" or most commonly, "paraprofessionals" (Morgan, 1976). Such a paraprofessional program was established at Santa Fe Community College, Gainesville, Florida in 1970 and designated as the Human Services Program (HSP).

The purpose of the HSP is to provide intensive training in human relations, general helping skills, psychopathology, and different approaches to counseling. The two most important assumptions underlying the program are: (1) that the single most critical resource a person has to bring to the helping situation is himself as an open, sensitive, caring human being; and (2) that the most effective learning takes place in situations in which a person is actively working in the area of study.

The core skills taught are those which deal with those competencies that should be possessed by persons working in a human services agency. These skills include interviewing and therapeutic skills, knowledge of community resources and community dynamics, process recording and psychopathology. Fieldwork competencies deal with skills related to working directly with people and the student's ability to apply the knowledge he has obtained. Fieldwork skills include conducting on-going counseling and in-take interviews, working with groups, case management activities, client advocacy, outreach and any other activities that human service agencies require of their counselors.

In addition to their other courses, students are required to take a minimum of 18 hours of general education, including mathematics, science, communications, humanities and social and behavioral sciences. At the completion of this curriculum students are awarded an A.S. degree in Human Services work.

Counselor Behavior Variables

Rogers (1957) presented an organized theoretical formulation in which he hypothesized that three characteristics of the counselor, when adequately communicated to the client, are both necessary and sufficient conditions for constructive personality and behavior change. These are: (1) empathic understanding of the client by the counselor; (2)

unconditional positive regard for the client by the counselor; and (3) the genuineness or self-congruence of the counselor in the counseling relationship. The improvement of the counselor's position and professional status is the major stimulus for the present research.

To achieve a more effective level of counseling Truax and Carkhuff (1967) have elaborated upon the position of Rogers and sought to describe the process of effective counseling and/or interpersonal functioning more specifically. They proposed a model which brings together many theoretical orientations:

> Despite the bewildering array of divergent theories and the difficulty in translating concepts from the language of one theory to that of another, several common threads weave their way through almost every major theory of psychotherapy and counseling, including psychoanalytic, client centered, behavioristic, and many of the more eclectic and derivative theories. In one way or another all have emphasized the importance of the therapist's ability to be integrated, mature, genuine, authentic or congruent in his relationship to the patient. They have all stressed the importance of the therapist's ability to provide a non-threatening, trusting, safe or secure atmosphere by acceptance, non-possessive warmth, unconditional positive regard or love. Finally, virtually all theories of psychotherapy emphasize that for the therapist to be helpful he must be accurately empathic, be "with" the client, be understanding, or grasp the patient's meaning.
> These sets of characteristics can for lack of better words be termed accurate empathy, non-possessive warmth and genuineness. (Truax & Carkhuff, 1967, p. 25)

The evidence of a growing number of studies (Carkhuff, 1968; Truax & Carkhuff, 1967: Luborsky, Auerback, Chandler, Cohen, & Backrach, 1971) strongly indicate that therapists who exhibit more of the aforementioned conditions are significantly more helpful in terms of client growth, while those who provide low levels of these conditions are actually harmful.

Meditation

One technique that shows great promise for enhancing the positive personality characteristics of counselors is meditation. Meditation is increasingly becoming a subject of empirical study. Research in meditation indicates that behaviors derived from such practices are compatible with and facilitative of counselor behaviors as taught in the traditional and developing schools of counseling and psycho-therapy (Keefe, 1973).

Investigations of meditation have yielded interesting results. A variety of psychological and physiological changes are reported in research studies cited by the Tran-scendental Meditation Society and reviewed by Bloomfield, Cain and Jaffe (1975), Kanellakos and Ferguson (1973), Kanellakos and Lukas (1974), Wallace (1970a, 1970b), and Wallace, Benson and Wilson (1971).

Of most interest to psychotherapists is that meditation has been found to be productive of enhanced empathic ability (Keefe, 1976) and correlates highly with measures of enhanced interpersonal functioning (Lesh, 1970).

A technique of meditation that is highly valuable for future research and which has been adapted for use in the present study is one described by Benson (1975) called the Relaxation Response (RR). This method is best suited for research because it is well standardized and therefore makes possible further studies under uniform conditions. In addition, it is easily learned so that experience is developed after only a short period of training. Furthermore, learning the technique does not involve adherence to any specific religion, belief system or life style.

Hypotheses

The present researcher agrees that accurate empathy, genuineness and respect are necessary characteristics of effective counselors and that any process which increases these characteristics in an individual is contributing to the development of a more effective counselor. This is true whether the candidate is a paraprofessional or a fully certified professional. Furthermore, meditation appears to be a technique which can contribute to counselor effectiveness by enhancing the positive personality characteristics mentioned above.

On the basis of these assumptions, the following hypotheses were tested. The hypothesis for the study related to four dimensions for measuring the subject's ability to relate interpersonally and one dimension measuring the subject's level of self-actualization. Three hypotheses (one major and two minor) were concerned with each of the dimensions. The major hypotheses were statements of no difference between groups. The minor hypotheses were statements of no difference within each treatment group.

Hypothesis 1: Self-Actualization

H_1 There will be no significant difference between subjects in the RR* and NRR** groups on self-actualization as measured by the Personal Orientation Inventory.

   H_{1A} There will be no significant gain in self-actualization for subjects in the RR group.

   H_{1B} There will be no significant gain in self-actualization for subjects in the NRR group.

Hypothesis 2: Affective/Cognitive

H_2 There will be no significant difference in gain between subjects in the RR and NRR groups on the feeling level of the responses to the clients.

   H_{2A} There will be no significant gain in feeling level of the responses to their clients for subjects in the RR group.

   H_{2B} There will be no significant gain in feeling level in the responses to their clients for subjects in the NRR group.

Hypothesis 3: Understanding/Nonunderstanding

H_3 There will be no significant difference in gain between subjects in the RR and the NRR groups in understanding of client responses.

   H_{3A} There will be no significant gain in understanding of client responses for subjects in the RR group.

---

*RR - trained in Relaxation Response (experimental group).
**NRR - no training in Relaxation Response (control group).

H_{3B} There will be no significant gain in understanding of client responses for subjects in the NRR group.

Hypothesis 4: Specific/Nonspecific

H_4 There will be no significant difference in gain between subjects in the RR and the NRR groups in the degree of specificity of responses to their clients.

H_{4A} There will be no significant gain in the degree of specificity of responses to clients for subjects in the RR group.

H_{4B} There will be no significant gain in the degree of specificity of responses to clients for subjects in the NRR group.

Hypothesis 5: Exploratory/Nonexploratory

H_5 There will be no significant difference in gain between subjects in the RR and the NRR groups in ability to give responses that lead clients to further self-exploration.

H_{5A} There will be no significant gain in ability to give responses that lead clients to further self-exploration for subjects in the RR group.

H_{5B} There will be no significant gain in ability to give responses that lead clients to further self-exploration for subjects in the NRR group.

Need for the Study

The ideas generated by Carkhuff and Truax have been of great value to the field of counseling in describing how the effective helper interacts with his client. However, Bergin (1966), Carkhuff (1969a, 1969b), and Truax and Carkhuff (1967) have all advocated the need for more research investigating ways of developing more positive personality characteristics of counselors.

The research herein presented is an attempt to assist in the fulfillment of the need for aiding counselors in providing the therapeutic and facilitative conditions requisite of client growth by enhancing personal functioning through meditation.

CHAPTER II

REVIEW OF RELATED RESEARCH

The review of pertinent research is divided into the following four areas: (1) Counselor-offered conditions contributing to client growth; (2) Facilitative condition and Personality; (3) Psychological effects of meditation, and (4) Theory of meditation.

Counselor-offered Conditions, Personality and Client Growth

In 1952 and 1961 Eysenck published research which seemed to deny the value of counseling and psychotherapy (Eysenck, 1952, 1961). These controversial articles caused those who were convinced of the benefits of counseling to try to find ways to show its effectiveness. Part of what they found was that there were some factors that could be isolated which distinguished effective from ineffective therapists. These ingredients Rogers calls the "necessary and sufficient conditions" for therapeutic change (Rogers, 1961). These necessary and sufficient conditions have become the basis for the scales measuring counselor effectiveness that Truax developed (Truax, 1961b, 1962a, 1962b).

Since the early 1960's Truax, Carkhuff and others have conducted research on therapist and client variables that have accounted for positive outcomes in therapy (Truax & Carkhuff, 1967; Carkhuff, 1966; Carkhuff, 1969a; Carkhuff & Berenson, 1967).

The Truax and Carkhuff research findings can be summarized as follows:

(1) Individuals possessing such personal character-istics as empathic understanding, nonpossessive warmth and genuineness can effect positive changes in clients. They can also rapidly develop more sophisticated therapeutic skills.

(2) Counselors who have the facilitative inter-personal qualities effect therapeutic changes without fully understanding the complexities of personality dynamics.

(3) Lengthy professional training is not a pre-requisite for effective functioning as a therapist.

(4) Paraprofessionals with limited training can be just as effective as professionals in facilitat-ing client change over relatively short periods of time.

Piaget, Berenson, and Carkhuff (1967) found that high-functioning therapists elicited higher levels of client self-exploration than did moderate-functioning therapists.

The higher the initial level of client self-exploration, the more elevated it becomes in the presence of a high-functioning therapist, whereas the moderate to poor therapist had his most deleterious effects on clients with initially low levels of self-exploration. When therapists intentionally lowered their levels of functioning during the middle third of the interview, the self-exploration of those clients of moderate-functioning therapists were more seriously lowered and the moderate-functioning therapists appeared less able to reestablish the earlier exhibited level of facilitative conditions.

Cannon and Pierce (1968) designed a two-way study to check on the effect of lowered and heightened facilitative conditions. The therapists saw three patients in a 45 minute interview. Group I therapists offered Hi-Low-Hi conditions and Group II therapists offered Low-Hi-Low conditions. Results indicate that the clients explored themselves more deeply ($p<.05$) when the therapists offered high-level conditions.

Holder (1968) found that high-functioning helpers have clients who engage in significantly fewer ($p<.05$) topics and engage in each topic for approximately 20 minutes. The study compared nine high rated versus nine low rated interviewers.

In studying the effects of these conditions in other settings Aspy (1965) found that students receiving relatively high levels of empathic understanding, warmth and genuineness from teachers gained significantly in reading achievement ($p<.01$). Truax and Tatum (1966) found that observer ratings of facilitative behavior of teachers were significantly correlated with increased socialization and adjustment of their students. Thus, the above mentioned conditions seem to be important for facilitative teacher-child relationships as well as counselor-client relationships.

Facilitative Conditions and Personality

A few research investigations have attempted to study the relationships between particular personality characteristics of counselors and their ability to offer the therapeutic conditions previously mentioned.

Bergin and Solomon (1963) found that the Depression ($p<.05$) and Psychasthenia ($p<.01$) scale of the Minnesota Multiphasic Personality Inventory (MMPI) correlated negatively with ratings of therapist empathy. The Consistency, Intraception and Order Scale of the Edwards Personal Preference Schedule (EPPS) were negatively correlated and Dominance and Change were positively correlated with empathy. All correlations were statistically significant ($p<.05$).

Foulds (1967) found significant positive relationships between self-actualization measures, the Personal
Orientation Inventory (POI), and counselor trainees' ability
to offer conditions of empathy and genuineness at the end
of their practicum. This research found six POI scales
related to empathy and 10 to 12 scales related to
genuineness. Therefore, as measured by these scales,
positive mental health is related to the provision of a
positive therapeutic condition.

Truax and Carkhuff (1967, pp. 233-235) cite the
unpublished findings of Truax, Silber, and Wargo (1966)
of the correlation between counselor offered conditions of
empathic understanding, positive regard and genuineness
with EPPS scores. In this study the MMPI and the EPPS were
administered to 16 graduate students in counseling before
and after experiencing an integrated didactic and experiential approach to training (Truax & Carkhuff, 1967).
Tape recorded counseling sessions were made early and late
in the training program and were then evaluated with respect
to the trainees' ability to communicate empathic understanding, positive regard, and genuineness to their clients.
Students showing high ability to offer these conditions
were then compared with students of lower ability in
demonstrating these conditions. Counselors showing the
greatest ability to provide the therapeutic conditions were

initially lower on the Order, Intraception, and Deference scales of the EPPS than counselors who showed little or no gain in ability to offer the therapeutic conditions.

The counselors who scored higher initially in the Change and Autonomy scales scored even higher on these scales by the end of the training program. Truax, Silber and Wargo's findings were highly consistent with the findings of the previously cited Bergin and Solomon study.

The data gathered from the studies cited above suggest that the counselor's ability to offer high levels of therapeutic or facilitative conditions in a counseling relationship may be dependent on the well-being and personal adequacy of the counselor. These studies have indicated that counselors who are anxious, defensive, conflicted or personally inadequate are least likely to facilitate constructive behavior change in their clients. Conversely, there is a positive relationship between the personal adequacy, authenticity or self-actualization of the counselor and his ability to facilitate constructive change in his clients.

These studies emphasize the direct effects of the helper's interpersonal level of functioning on the helpee. According to Carkhuff's model, the degree to which the helping person offers high levels of empathy, positive regard, and genuineness is related directly to the degree

of the client's ability to internalize these facilitative
conditions into his own personal life. In addition, the
degree to which the action-oriented helpful counselor is
freely, spontaneously, and deeply himself, disclosing of
himself, actively confronting himself and the client,
being in the moment, and taking concrete courses of action
is directly related to the helpee's ability to apply these
same facilitative activities in his own life situation.

Counselor Verbal Responses Approach

Attempts to measure counselor effectiveness through
types and levels of verbal responses given by the counselor
are probably the most widely researched of all the different system of measuring counselor effectiveness. Carkhuff,
Truax, Berenson, and Rogers have been leading researchers
in this area. Their research deals primarily with relating
a set of interpersonal core factors to client gain. These
factors are empathy, unconditional positive regard, con-
gruency, and concreteness. Effectiveness of communication
of these relationship factors is measured through scales
that assess the effectiveness of counselor responses on
those dimensions.

In his model for effective therapy Carkhuff offers
several propositions concerning the effect of facilitative
helper dimensions on the client-counselor interaction. A
review of his two propositions and corollaries seems appropriate as the interactional scale used in this study closely

relates to that used by Carkhuff. In <u>Helping and Human Relations, Volume One</u>, he supports the following statements with a wide variety of research evidence.

<u>Proposition I</u>. The degree to which the helping person offers high levels of facilitative conditions in response to the expressions of the person seeking help, is related directly to the degree to which the person seeking help engages in processes to constructive change or gain.

Corollary I. The degree to which the helping person offers high levels of empathic understanding of the helpee's world is related directly to the degree to which the helpee is able to understand himself and others.

Corollary II. The degree to which the helping person communicates high levels of respect and warmth for the helpee and his world is related directly to the degree to which the helpee is able to respect and direct warm feelings toward himself and others.

Corollary III. The degree to which the helper is helpful in guiding exploration to specific feelings and content is related directly to the degree to which the helpee is able to make concrete his own problem areas.

Corollary IV. The degree to which the helper is responsively genuine in his relationship with the helpee is related to the degree to which the helpee is able to be responsively genuine in his relationship with himself and others.

<u>Proposition II</u>. The degree to which the helping person initiates action-oriented dimensions in a helping relationship is directly related to the degree to which the person seeking help engages in processes that lead to constructive change or growth.

Corollary I. The degree to which the helper can be freely, spontaneously and deeply himself, including the disclosing of significant information about himself when appropriate, is

directly related to the degree to which the
helpee is able to be genuine and self-
disclosing in appropriate relationships.

Corollary II. The degree to which the helper
actively confronts the helpee and himself is
directly related to the degree to which the
helpee is able to confront himself and others.

Corollary III. The degree to which the helper
both acts and directs the actions of the
helpee immediately in the present in the
relationship between helper and helpee is related to the helpee's ability to act with
immediacy and later to direct the actions of
others.

Corollary IV. The degree to which the helper
can make concrete a course of constructive
action is related to the degree to which the
helpee can go on to make concrete courses of
action for himself and others. (Carkhuff,
1969, pp. 84-90)

These statements emphasize the direct effects of the
helper's interpersonal level of function on the helpee.
According to Carkhuff's model, the degree to which the
helping person offers high levels of empathy, warmth, respect, concreteness, and genuineness is related directly to
the degree of the client's ability to internalize these
facilitative conditions into his own personal life. In
addition, the degree to which the action-oriented helpful
counselor is freely, spontaneously, and deeply himself,
disclosing of himself, actively confronting himself and the
client, being with the moment, and making concrete courses
of action is directly related to the helpee's ability to
apply these same facilitative activities in his own life
situation.

The Counselor Verbal Response Scale (CVRS) has been found to have a .40 positive correlation with the Carkhuff scales (Schauble, Pierce, & Resnikoff, 1976). Additionally, it has been found to be more sensitive to small gains in interpersonal level of functioning and thus more appropriate for measuring relatively short-term counselor trainee progress (Schauble, Pierce, & Resnikoff, 1976).

Psychological Effects of Meditation

The research available on meditation suggests that the technique may be able to increase the degree of positive personal characteristics needed by professional helpers. These behaviors include enhanced awareness of one's own feelings, the ability to hold cognitive processes in abeyance, enhanced perception, and increased present centeredness. The purpose of this section is to examine some of the relevant investigations of meditation.

Much of meditation research has been conducted by the members of the Transcendental Meditation Society (Bloomfield et al., 1975); therefore, these studies will be reviewed first.

Transcendental Meditation

Most of the studies investigating the psychological effects of Transcendental Meditation (TM) have used paper-and-pencil tests. Some attention has been devoted to the effects of TM on self-actualization as measured by the POI. In the first such study (Seeman, Nidich, & Banta, 1972) meditators and nonmeditators were administered the POI two months apart. For the TM group, the first administration took place two days prior to instruction in TM. There were no differences between these groups on the first administration. But upon retesting the meditators scored significantly higher ($p < .05$) than nonmeditators on 6 of the 12 scales (inner directedness, self-actualizing value, spontaneity, self-regard, acceptance of aggression, and capacity for intimate contact). In a second study using the same design Nidich, Seeman, and Dreskin (1973) found similar differences in 10 of the 12 POI scales.

The differences found in these two studies were thought to have been influenced by expectancy, that is, the experimental subjects expected to experience positive personality changes from the practice of meditation, whereas nonmeditators had no such expectation of change. Hjelle (1974), in order to test for this possibility, compared two groups of experienced meditators (meditating average of 22.6 months) and novice meditators who were tested a week prior to being instructed in TM. Experienced meditators scored higher on 7 of the 12 POI scales (inner directedness, time competence, spontaneity, self-regard, self-actualizing value, feeling reactivity, and capacity for intimate contact. The findings of Seeman et al. (1972) were supported by this study on five scales (inner directedness, spontaneity, self-regard, self-actualizing value, and capacity for intimate contact). This suggests that expectancy may not have made any significant difference in accounting for the observed changes.

Russie (1975) suggested that expectancy may be at least a minor factor in the changes in the POI scores as a result of TM. Meditators and nonmeditators were tested five months apart, meditators having been first tested two days prior to learning TM. After five months, meditators scored significantly higher than nonmeditators on seven scales (inner directedness, time competence, self-actualizing value, feeling reactivity, spontaneity, self-acceptance, and capacity for intimate contact). Changes on four of these scales (inner directedness, self-actualizing value, spontaneity, and capacity for intimate contact) replicated the findings of both Seeman et al. (1972) and Hjelle (1974). However, as determined by correlation between subjects' pretest expectation scores and actual pre- and posttest differences, a significant positive relationship (p<.04) was found between prospective meditators' expectations of positive changes and the results achieved in six of the POI scales. Thus, while some of the changes in the POI do appear to be a result of practicing TM, and are replicable, they do not seem to have resulted entirely from expectancy. Apparently expectation of change may account for at least some of the variance in these differences.

Drennen and Chermol (in press) noted that initial studies of the effects of TM on self-actualization (Seeman et al., 1972; Nidich et al., 1973) did not control for possible expectancy or placebo effect. That is, meditators were not compared with nonmeditators who followed other practices of regularly sitting quietly. These early studies compared three groups: meditators, nonmeditators (who were told to relax following a relaxation training twice a day for 20 minute periods) and no treatment controls. The POI was administered prior to instruction and again one month later. Subjects in all groups showed positive changes on the second administration of the POI: on 5 scales for the control group, 6 scales for the TM group, and 9 scales for the relaxation group. These results were interpreted as indicating (a) that placebo effects need to be taken into account in TM research, and (b) that other relaxation techniques may produce changes similar to those resulting from TM.

Dick and Ragland (1973) administered the POI eight weeks apart to three groups of subjects who (a) learned TM, (b) received individual counseling and learned TM, or (c) received individual counseling and rested quietly for 15 minutes twice each day. Subjects in the latter two groups were drawn from individuals seeking treatment at a counseling center and were randomly assigned to groups. Thus, expectancy was controlled in that subjects in all three groups expected some improvement, and the relaxation variable was controlled by having control subjects rest twice daily. The authors predicted that scores of the counseling plus TM groups would be higher than for the group practicing TM alone, which in turn, would be higher than the counseling with rest group. This hypothesis was supported (p<.05) for the time competence and inner directedness scales. It appears, then, that TM facilitates certain changes measured by the POI to a greater extent than expectancy or rest alone can account for.

Research to date indicates that the regular practice of TM certainly results in significantly positive changes in self-actualization as measured by the POI. However, it is quite possible that there may be other relaxation techniques which produce similar changes. Transcendental meditation has not been shown to be unique in its effects on self-actualization as measured by the POI.

Relaxation Response

Another method of meditation which lends itself well to research is that described by Benson. It is called the Relaxation Response (RR). Beary and Benson (1974) have provided evidence that RR is effective in eliciting the relaxation response as defined by Benson and his colleagues (Benson, 1975; Benson, Beary, & Carol, 1974; Wallace, Benson, & Wilson, 1971). Seventeen subjects, each serving as his own control, learned RR by reading instructions from a sheet of paper. Subjects were novices at this technique. Expectancy was minimized by telling subjects that only the physiology of relaxation was being investigated. During the experiment, subjects practiced RR during 1 of 5 consecutive periods of 12 minutes each. During control periods subjects either sat quietly and read material of neutral emotional content or sat with eyes closed. Subjects were randomly assigned to two sequences. Oxygen consumption, carbon dioxide production and respiration rate were measured. All three were significantly lower during the RR period than during control periods. These results were interpreted as indicating changes resulting from RR.

While the research on the effects of RR has been very limited, especially with regard to psychological data, initial findings suggest that the physiological and emotional states produced by RR are similar to if not the same as those associated with TM. Further, the regular practice of RR may have beneficial long-term effects. This new technique offers the opportunity for more highly controlled studies of meditation.

Meditation in Theory

Three theories, two psychological and one physiological, have been put forth to account for the effects of meditation.

Psychoanalytic Derepression

Initiates to TM (and to certain other forms of meditation) are repeatedly reminded of the need for effortlessness.

That is, during meditation extraneous thoughts are not to
be resisted any more than they are to be attended to
closely; rather, such thoughts are to be allowed to occur
dispassionately. In practice, while a mantra is being repeated this effortless dealing with extraneous thoughts
amounts of noninterfering observation. Naranjo (1971) has
compared this observation to the activity of the second
witness (the therapist) to free associations of a patient
in the psychoanalytic situation. With repeated meditations,
resistance to the awareness of certain thoughts becomes
weakened, and such thoughts become increasingly spontaneous.

Shaffii (1973) has compared the meditation and psychoanalytic processes in detail. Two major events are common
to both. The reexperiencing of psychic traumas during
meditation frees psychic energy for present uses. This
amounts to bringing repressed thoughts into consciousness
and transcending the conflicts related to them. The repetition of such events leads gradually to a controlled regres-
sion to a nonverbal stage of development, at which point
traumatic experiences can be resolved internally at a level
deeper than verbal or cognitive processes permit. The major
difference between psychoanalysis and meditation is that the
former emphasizes verbalization and the latter silence. The
therapeutic aspects of both processes are seen to be the
same.

Generalized Desensitization

A second theory, behavioral in nature, is quite compatible with the first. Goleman (1971, 1974), noting the similarity between the relaxation states produced by both meditation and relaxation training, has compared meditation with systematic desensitization. In the latter, a hierarchy of images troublesome to a patient is presented to him by a therapist while he is relaxed, beginning with the least anxiety-producing images and ending with the most troublesome. Anxiety responses are thereby inhibited by the association of relaxation with stimuli. In meditation, the contents of the mind (both verbalizations and imagery) are presented to consciousness in a self-regulated manner while the meditator is relaxed. As troublesome thoughts occur, anxiety is inhibited by the association of relaxation with such thoughts. While this occurs in a less systematic manner than in desensitization, the hierarchy is optimally salient to the individual. Meditation is seen as a slower and less efficient means to the same end, but perhaps a more thorough one in that items in the hierarchy are not limited to those selected by therapist and patient.

The Relaxation Response (RR)

A third theory, compatible with both of the above theories, is based on the physiological correlates of meditation. Benson (1975) and Benson et al. (1974) have theorized that the physiological changes associated with meditation constitute "an integrated hypothalamic

response which results in generalized decreased sympathetic
nervous system activity, and perhaps also increased para-
sympathetic activity" (Benson et al., 1974, p. 37). This
relaxation response is the counterpart of the flight-or-
fight response of extreme arousal. The latter is also an
integrated response, mediated by the sympathetic nervous
system and characterized by increased arousal and body
metabolism, which is elicited by and prepares an organism
for dealing with a threatening situation or set of stimuli.

Because civilized man is socially reinforced for
inhibiting literal fight-or-flight responses, the repeated
elicitation of the fight-or-flight response in varying
degrees results in the accumulation of stress at a physiological level, and probably at other levels as well. A
person thus may become less efficient with time due to ever-
accumulating stress. The regular elicitation of the
relaxation response, which TM and other forms of meditation
provide, serves both to release accumulated stresses and
to prevent further accumulation. This may result in the
alleviation and prevention of physical, mental, and emotional
symptoms that are produced by stress.

French and Tupin (1973, 1974) and Benson (1975a and b)
have developed procedures designed to elicit the relaxation
response in a manner similar to that of TM and other forms
of meditation. The latter procedure is the only one to
have been researched in a controlled manner.

Benson (1975b) reported that his technique for eliciting the relaxation response was developed by comparing the various practices of meditation, yoga, prayer, and secular relaxation practices. Four essential components were found to be common to these practices: (a) a mental device consisting of some constant stimulus upon which attention is focused; (b) a passive attitude (i.e., not trying to relax and not worrying about whether the technique is being practiced correctly); (c) decreased muscle tonus, which necessitates a posture conducive to relaxation; and (d) a quiet environment in which outside stimuli are minimal. The procedure for eliciting the relaxation response, as described by Benson (1975), consists of having a person sit quietly in a comfortable position, close his eyes, relax all the body muscles (beginning with the feet and progressing upward to the face), and once relaxation is attained, repeat silently to himself the word "ONE" in conjunction with each respiratory exhalation.

Elements of Meditation

Beary and Benson (1974) have provided evidence that this technique of meditation is effective in eliciting the relaxation response as defined by Benson and his colleagues (Benson, 1975; Benson et al., 1975; Wallace et al., 1971). Seventeen subjects, each serving as his own control, learned RR by reading instructions from a sheet of paper. Prior to being studied, practice had been limited to one hour, so

that subjects were relative novices at the technique.
Expectancy was minimized by telling subjects only that the
physiology of relaxation was being investigated. During the
experiment, subjects practiced the RR during 1 of 5 consecutive periods of 12 minutes each. During control periods,
subjects either sat quietly and read material of neutral
emotional content or sat with eyes closed. Subjects were
randomly assigned to two sequences. Oxygen consumption,
carbon dioxide production, and respiration rate were measured. All three were significantly lower during the RR
period than during control periods, and sitting with eyes
closed resulted in no differences from sitting and reading.

There is also evidence that the regular practice of RR
may have long-term physiological effects. Benson (1975b;
Beary & Benson, 1974) reported that the regular practice of
RR has been found to be associated with decreased blood
pressure in hypertensive patients and increased blood pressure in hypotensive patients. Benson, Alexander, and
Feldman (1975) found that the regular practice of RR after
four weeks reduced premature ventricular contractions in
patients with ischaemic heart disease during both wakeful-
ness and sleep.

The previously cited research of Benson et al. (1975)
and Benson et al. (1974) have provided evidence that this
technique of meditation is effective in eliciting the relaxation response as defined by Benson (1975). The results of

these studies were interpreted as indicating changes
resulting from the RR were similar to those resulting from
TM.

CHAPTER III

EXPERIMENTAL DESIGN AND PROCEDURES

This chapter discusses the experimental design used in the study and the major considerations involved. It includes a description of the training program, the study population, the hypotheses advanced, and the criterion instruments employed. In addition, the chapter provides an explanation of experimental procedures used in the investigation.

Experimental Design

This study employed the pretest-posttest control group design which included the following procedure:

1) the administration of a pretest to both groups;

2) administration of treatment to the experimental group, but not the control group, and

3) administration of a posttest to both groups.

Students were assigned to groups by means of their Personal Data Sheets collected during the orientation session. Each data sheet was numbered inconspicuously 1, 2, or 3 and distributed at the orientation session. Subjects whose sheets numbered 1 or 2 became the experimental group and those numbered 3 became the control group. However, these numbers were known only to the experimenter.

Population

A group of paraprofessional counselor students in their first term at the Santa Fe Community College Human Services Department was selected to be the subjects of this study. Out of a total of 36 students in the program, 28 volunteered initially. Two students dropped out of the Human Services program after two weeks and 4 dropped out of this study as subjects. The total number of subjects completing the study was 22 (see demographic data sheet, Appendix C).

Subjects' Demographic Data

Sex--The sexual composition of the groups are as follows: the experimental group had 9 females and 5 males. The control group had 4 females and 4 males.

Race--The experimental group had 11 whites and 3 blacks. The control group had 4 whites and 4 blacks.

Age--The figures for the total sample are: mean 26, range 19-52, mode 21, and median 23. The figures for the experimental group are: mean 27, range 19-52, mode 21, and median 23. The figures for the control group are: mean 24, range 19-38, mode 21, and median 22.

Marital status

	Experimental Group	Control Group
Single	42.8%	37.5%
Married	21.4%	12.5%
Separated, divorced or widowed	35.8%	50.0%

Research Instruments

The instruments used in this study were: the Personal Orientation Inventory (POI) (Shostrom, 1966) and the Counselor Verbal Response Scale (CVRS) (Kagan & Krathwohl, 1967).

Assessment of Self-Actualization

The psychological construct, "self-actualization," has been used by personality theorists such as Combs (1962), Maslow (1954, 1962), Rogers (1961), and others. Counselors, psychotherapists, personality theorists, and researchers have felt a need for a comprehensive measure of values and behavior seen to be of importance in the development of self-actualization. Shostrom (1964, 1966) developed the Personal Orientation Inventory (POI) to meet this need. Most diagnostic instruments have been developed for use with seriously disturbed psychiatric populations, and they attempt to provide measures of the subjects' pathology. This is a negative approach to personality assessment.

Shostrom (1966) appears to use the terms self-actualization, fully functioning, and positive mental health synonymously. A description of the POI is presented below.

Personal Orientation Inventory (POI)

The POI is an instrument developed by Shostrom (1964, 1966) which purports to provide a comprehensive measure of values believed to be of importance in the development of self-actualization or positive mental health. The POI consists of 150 two-choice paired-opposite statements of values, and scores are reported for 2 major scales and 10 secondary scales which purport to assess particular personality characteristics considered to be associated with self-actualization. The POI purports to assess a person's position on a continuum for each of the following personality variables.

Major Scales:

1. Time Competence (Tc): measures the degree to which one is "present" oriented.

2. Inner Direction (I): measures whether reactivity orientation is basically toward self or others.

Secondary Scales:

1. Self-Actualizing Values (SAV): measures affirmation of values held by self-actualizing persons.

2. Existentiality (Ex): measures ability to situationally or existentially react without rigid adherence to principles.

3. Feeling Reactivity (Fr): measures sensitivity of responsiveness to one's own needs and feelings.

4. Spontaneity (S): measures freedom to react spontaneously or to be oneself.

5. Self-Regard (Sr): measures affirmation of worth or strength.

6. Self-Acceptance (Sa): measures affirmation or acceptance of self in spite of weaknesses or deficiencies.

7. View of the Nature of Man (Nc): measures degree of the constructive view of the nature of man, masculinity, femininity.

8. Synergy (Sy): measures ability to be synergistic, to transcend dichotomies.

9. Acceptance of Aggression (A): measures ability to accept one's natural aggressiveness as opposed to defensiveness, denial, or repression of aggression.

10. Capacity for Intimate Contact (C): measures ability to develop contactful intimate relationships with other human beings, unencumbered by expectations and obligations.

The POI is essentially self-administered. The questions are printed in a reusable test booklet, and the examinee records his answers on a specially designed answer sheet. There is no time limit set for completion of the inventory. Testing time is usually about 30 to 40 minutes.

The POI was validated on 650 freshmen at Los Angeles State College, 75 members of a sensitivity training program at UCLA, and 15 school psychologists in a special training program. Retested after training, the latter two groups showed definite growth in inner directedness.

The POI was also tested on three other groups: 160 normal adults, 29 relatively self-actualized adults, and 34 relatively nonself-actualized adults nominated by the

clinical psychology societies of Orange and Los Angeles
Counties, California. The test does discriminate between
self-actualized and nonself-actualized persons on 11 of 12
scales according to Shostrom (1964).

Robert Knapp (1965) compared the POI with the Eysenck
Personality Inventory (EPI). The EPI measures neuroticism-
stability and extraversion-introversion. High- and low-
neurotic students were selected from 136 undergraduates on
the basis of their EPI and correlated with the POI. Low-
neurotic students tended toward self-actualization as did
extroverted students. The POI and EPI are from different
theoretical frames of reference but seem to be tapping a
common core. Shostrom and Knapp (1956) correlated the POI
with the Minnesota Multiphasic Personality Inventory (MMPI)
and found high correlations between the POI and the Social
I.E. (SI) and Depression (D) scales of the MMPI.

The POI manual gives high reliability correlations of
.91 to .93. An independent retest (50 week interval) study
gave a much more modest correlation of .55 for the Time
Competent (Tc) scale and .71 for the Inner Directed (I)
scale. The mean correlation for the subscales was .58.
Although this is not as high as would be desirable, it is
well within the range of reliability similarly established
for the Edwards Personal Preference Schedule and the MMPI
(Ilardi & May, 1968). On the basis of the above studies
it was felt that the POI would be a valid instrument for the
present research.

Counselor Verbal Response Scale (CVRS)

The CVRS purports to describe a counselor's response to client communication in terms of four dichotomized dimensions: (a) affective-cognitive; (b) understanding-nonunderstanding; (c) specific-nonspecific; (d) exploratory-nonexploratory. A fifth dimension, effective-noneffective, provides a global rating of the adequacy of each response which is made independently of the four descriptive ratings. For the purposes of this study the first four dimensions were used.

The unit of analysis was the verbal interaction between counselor and client represented by a client statement and counselor response. A counselor response is rated on each of the four dimensions of the rating scale, with every client-counselor interaction being judged independently of preceding units. In judging an individual response, the primary focus is on describing how the counselor responded to the verbal elements of the client's communication. The procedure is based upon the theories of Carl Rogers and theories and research of Truax and Carkhuff.

The CVRS consists of five forced choice dichotomous dimensions measuring the extent to which counselors are characterized by affective, understanding, specific, exploratory, and effective responses. The dimensions are defined as follows: An affective response is one which makes reference to or encourages some affective or feeling aspect of the client's communication while a cognitive response refers to the cognitive component of a client's statement; understanding refers to the counselor's ability to convey to the client his awareness of, and his sensitivity to, the client's feelings and concerns by attempting to deal with the core of his concerns rather than making vague responses or referring to peripheral concerns; exploratory responses encourage the client to explore his feelings and provide him with an opportunity to do so. Nonexploratory responses typically restrict the client's freedom to explore. The final dimension, effective-noneffective, is a global rating of overall effectiveness of a counselor's response in promoting client movement. A sample rating sheet can be found in Appendix B.

Inter-judge reliability was determined by applying Hoyt's analysis of variance technique to the ratings of two sets of judges who had rated the videotaped interviews of 50 inexperienced M.A. candidates in Counseling and Guidance at Michigan State University. Corresponding four minute segments were rated for 53 counselors (the post tape of one of the M.A. candidates was lost). Of the 53, 45 were M.S. candidates and 8 Ph.D. candidates, and they interviewed the same coached client. Because timed segments with unequal numbers of responses were used, ratings were converted to proportionate scores. Corresponding 20 response segments were rated for the remaining 10 counseling interviews.

Coefficients were obtained of average tape inter-judge
reliability of .84, .80, .79, .68, and .79 for the affective-
cognitive, understanding-nonunderstanding, specific-
nonspecific, exploratory-nonexploratory, and effective-
noneffective dimensions of the scale, respectively (Kagan &
Krathwohl, 1967).

These scales have been validated on 53 counselor education trainees. Forty-five of these trainees were M.A. candidates and 8 were Ph.D. candidates. Tapes of counseling
interviews from each of the trainees were collected and
rated using the CVRS. On each dimension of the scale signif-
icances (p<.01) were found between the responses of the Ph.D.
candidates and the M.A. candidates, with the former having
more responses rated as affective, understanding, specific,
exploratory, and effective (Kagan & Krathwohl, 1967). When
separate ratings were made of 10 counselors with M.A.'s
having some advanced training and counseling experience and
were compared to the ratings of the 53 trainees, the
response pattern of these counselors fell between those of
the M.A. and the Ph.D. candidates (Kagan & Krathwohl, 1967).
Other validation studies have been conducted by Kagan and
Krathwohl (1967, pp. 84-90).

The CVRS differs from other rating scales in that it
focuses on a series of individual client/counselor verbal
units (client statement . . . counselor response) during the
course of an interview, rather than on global ratings of

entire interviews or longer interview segments. Thus, the judge is required to describe every counselor response to a client's verbalization on each of the dimensions of the scale. After 20 counselor responses have been dichotomized on each dimension, totals are obtained. A sample rating record sheet can be found in Appendix B.

These scales have been validated through several studies presented by Kagan and Krathwohl (1967, pp. 84-90). Ratings in this scale have also been found to have a positive correlation with the Carkhuff scales (Schauble, Pierce & Resnikoff, 1976). These scales have also been validated in extensive process and outcome research in counseling and psychotherapy (Truax & Carkhuff, 1967). (Refer to Appendix B.)

Demographic Questionnaire

The demographic questionnaire or personal data sheet was intended to elicit personal information so that comparisons could be made between the two sample groups. This questionnaire was developed by the Human Services Department of Santa Fe Community College as a student data sheet. A sample of this form may be found in Appendix E.

Collection of Data

Initial Data

In an orientation session during the first week of classes for the winter semester 1977, 26 students volunteering for this study from the Human Services Program were pretested using the POI. At this time they also filled out a student data sheet. After completion of the POI the subjects were given a cassette tape and asked to make a 30 minute taped interview with a student in their class acting as a client who would share a problem with the subject acting as counselor. These tapes were made during class time with other students.

Selection and Training of Raters

Research on the selection of raters suggest that both raters' level of functioning and raters' training by a qualified professional are a significant influence on discrimination scores (Cannon & Carkhuff, 1969), and that persons functioning below minimal facilitation levels (level 3) would not be capable of accurate ratings. While the CVRS used in this research employs a dichotomous rating assignment, the training and rating procedure are essentially the same.

Four raters were selected from a group of graduate students in counseling psychology. Those individuals were functioning at above minimal levels of facilitative interaction, as judged by independent ratings of their own tapes as helpers. The training of the raters was conducted by a Counseling Psychologist, at the University of Florida's Counseling Center, who is experienced in using the process scales.

A pair of trained judges individually rated pre- and postinterview segments with respect to the CVRS. For the CVRS scale a 10 minute segment from each tape was selected. A 5 minute segment in the first half and a 5 minute segment in the second half of each counseling tape were used. Raters started rating the first response after the first minute of the interview. Then they advanced the tape to the middle and rated the following 5 minute segment.

Relaxation Response (RR) Training

All subjects attended a general meeting during the second week of the semester and the counseling tapes were collected. At this time the experimental group was told to remain for further training in the RR. Students in the control group met separately and were told they would learn the RR at the end of the semester.

The researcher then instructed the 14 experimental group subjects in the RR in three phases, in a manner similar to that described by Benson (1975).

Phase 1. Instructions:

Find a comfortable position. Close your eyes, Deeply relax your muscles as you repeat internally, "I relax my feet . . . I relax my calves . . . etc." Beginning at your feet and progressing up to your face--feet, calves, thighs, lower torso, chest, shoulders, neck, head. Allow them to remain deeply relaxed. Now breathe through your nose and feel your breathing.

(Students practiced this for 2 minutes.)

Phase 2. Instructions:

Sit comfortably with your eyes closed for a
moment . . . Open our eyes . . . Close the eyes
. . . Open the eyes . . . Were you aware of
thoughts during the silence? Did you notice
how easily and naturally they came? This is
how easily you should think of the sound "So"
as you breathe in and "Hum" as you breathe out.
Now close your eyes again and begin repeating the
sound "So" each time you breathe in and "Hum"
each time you breathe out. Slowly open the eyes.
(Student practiced this for 5 minutes.)

Phase 3. Instructions:

This is the way to do the RR. Remember, don't
resist thoughts or sounds, but when they occur,
gently allow your mind to return to the sound
"So" when breathing in and "Hum" when breathing
out. Remember to wait about half a minute with
eyes closed before beginning to practice and take
a couple of minutes to open your eyes after you
finish. Are there any questions? (At this point
questions that may arise are answered and subjects are given an opportunity to discuss their
experience with RR.)

Before the training session ended subjects were given written instructions to take with them (Appendix A) on how to bring forth the relaxation response.

Students were then reminded to practice the RR daily for the duration of the semester and were given a calendar to record the time and days they practiced (Appendix C).

Posttest

A date and time were set for posttesting in 10 weeks. At that time all subjects were given the POI for the second time. Subjects were given a second cassette tape to record a posttest counseling tape to be submitted the following week.

Upon receiving all the tapes, the control group was trained during the last week of the semester in the RR in the manner described above.

CVRS Data Collection

At the conclusion of the semester all pre- and post-tapes which had been collected by the experimenter were sent to the University of Florida Counseling Center for analyses on the CVRS scale by a trained set of raters (see section on Selection and Training of Raters, page 41 above) and subsequently returned to the experimenter.

Statistical Design

The criterion instruments were administered to the subjects in both experimental and control groups prior to

and after the first semester of training in the Human
Services Program. Analysis of the POI score employed the
Mann-Whitney U test. The Mann-Whitney U test may be used
to test whether two independent groups have been drawn from
the same population. This is one of the most powerful of
the nonparametric tests, and it is a most useful alternative
to the parametric "t" test when the researcher wishes to
avoid the "t" test's assumptions, or when the measurement
in the research is weaker than interval scaling (Siegel,
1956). However, for purposes of comparing the results, the
traditional "t" test was also made on the POI scores and
those results are also shown. The analysis of the CVRS data
employs the "t" test as well as cross-tabular analysis of
the CVRS scores converted to percentage figures.

CHAPTER IV
RESULTS OF THE STUDY

The purpose of this study was to investigate the effect of the Relaxation Response on the personality characteristics of paraprofessional counselors. In the first part of this chapter, the analyses of the data relevant to the hypothesis are reported. In the second part of the chapter, additional analyses are summarized.

Two instruments were used to measure and evaluate 16 variables in a pre-post test design. Five major hypotheses and 10 minor hypotheses were concerned with each of the variables. The major hypotheses were statements of no difference between groups. The minor hypotheses were statements of no difference within each treatment group. The Mann-Whitney U was used to test measures of Self-Actualization as was the Wilcoxon Signed-Rank Statistic and the "t" test statistic. The "t" test statistic was used to test the significance of changes in proportion of facilitative responses on the CVRS.

Testing of the Hypothesis

Hypothesis 1: Self-Actualization

Hypothesis H_1: There will be no significant difference in gain in self-actualization between subjects in the RR (experimental) and in the NRR (control) groups as measured by the POI.

A summary of the analysis of the posttest POI scores relevant to this hypothesis is found in Table 1. Because of the significant gains ($p<.05$) made in five of the scales (Other, Inner, Existentiality, Spontaneity, Self-Acceptance, and Acceptance of Aggression) the hypothesis H_1 was rejected.

Hypothesis H_{1A}: There will be no significant gain in self-actualization for RR (experimental) group subjects.

A summary of the analysis of the Experimental Group pretest vs posttest scores relevant to this hypothesis is found in Table 2. Because of the significant gains in the Inner Directed, Spontaneity, Self-Regard and the Self-Acceptance scales (see Table 2 for the relevant confidence levels) hypothesis H_{1A} was rejected.

Hypothesis H_{1B}: There will be no significant gain in self-actualization for subjects in the NRR (control) group.

A summary of the analysis of the Control Group pretest vs posttest POI scores relevant to this hypothesis is found in Table 3. Because of the lack of significant gains in the scales hypothesis H_{1B} was accepted.

Table 1
Analysis of Posttest POI Scores
Control vs Experimental Groups

POI symbol**	Control mean	S.D.	Experimental mean	S.D.	Mean difference	U*	Significance
Ti	7.88	4.27	6.00	3.08	-1.88	38	NS
Tc	15.13	4.27	17.01	3.08	1.88	38	NS
O	46.13	9.51	34.87	13.33	-11.26	30	p<.05 Exp.<Cont.
I	79.25	9.48	91.94	13.31	12.69	29	p<.05 Exp.>Cont.
SAV	20.00	2.23	19.93	2.93	- .07	49	NS
Ex	17.38	3.66	22.15	5.40	4.77	27	p<.05 Exp.>Cont.
Fr	15.75	2.62	17.57	2.98	1.82	32.5	NS
S	12.38	2.77	14.72	1.81	2.34	31	p<.05 Exp.>Cont.
Sr	11.13	2.36	12.87	2.28	1.74	35	NS
Sa	13.75	2.56	17.86	3.09	-4.11	17	p<.05 Exp.>Cont.
Nc	11.25	2.72	12.29	1.51	1.04	45	NS
Sy	6.25	.94	6.72	1.09	0.47	49.5	NS
A	14.75	1.89	16.51	3.64	1.76	32	NS
C	17.38	4.40	20.37	3.82	2.99	33.5	NS

*Mann-Whitney U.
**See Figure 1 for symbol description.

Table 2
Analysis of Experimental Group
Pretest vs Posttest POI Scores

POI symbol**	Pretest mean	S.D.	Posttest mean	S.D.	Mean difference	W*	Significance
Ti	6.21	2.77	6.00	3.08	-0.21	42	NS
Tc	16.80	2.77	17.01	3.08	0.21	42	NS
O	39.94	9.60	34.87	13.33	-5.07	29	NS
I	85.43	9.55	91.94	13.31	6.51	26.5	NS
SAV	20.51	2.79	19.93	2.93	-0.58	22	NS
Ex	20.79	3.71	22.15	5.40	1.36	30.5	NS
Fr	16.86	2.72	17.57	2.98	0.71	27	NS
S	13.79	1.67	14.72	1.81	0.93	21	NS
Sr	11.87	2.21	12.87	2.28	1.00	13	p<.05 Post>Pre
Sa	14.79	2.72	17.86	3.09	3.07	20	p<.05 Post>Pre
Nc	12.29	1.54	12.29	1.51	0	38.5	NS
Sy	6.86	1.09	6.72	1.09	- .14	8	NS
A	15.87	2.73	16.51	3.64	0.64	40.5	NS
C	19.16	2.43	20.37	3.82	1.21	24.5	NS

*Wilcoxon Signed-Rank Statistic.
**See Figure 1 for symbol description.

Table 3
Analysis of Control Group
Pretest vs Posttest POI Scores

POI symbol**	Pretest mean	S.D.	Posttest mean	S.D.	Mean difference	W*	Significance
Ti	7.88	3.13	7.88	4.27	0	10.5	NS
Tc	15.13	3.13	15.13	4.27	0	10.5	NS
O	43.75	6.99	46.13	9.51	2.38	12	NS
I	78.00	8.03	79.25	9.48	1.25	10.5	NS
SAV	18.75	3.88	20.00	2.23	1.25	5	NS
Ex	17.75	4.31	17.38	3.66	-0.37	9	NS
Fr	15.63	1.37	15.75	2.62	0.12	18	NS
S	12.38	1.64	12.38	2.77	0	14	NS
Sr	11.50	2.28	11.13	2.36	-0.37	10.5	NS
Sa	14.13	3.01	13.75	2.57	-0.38	6	NS
Nc	8.75	2.32	11.25	2.72	2.50	1.5	NS
Sy	6.50	.83	6.25	.94	- .25	5	NS
A	15.88	1.26	14.75	1.89	1.13	7	NS
C	17.88	2.56	17.38	4.40	- .50	12.5	NS

*Wilcoxon Signed-Rank Statistic.
**See Figure 1 for symbol description.

At this point it should be noted that the Mann-Whitney U showed no significant differences between the pretest POI scores of the control and experimental groups with the single exception of the scale, Nature of Man, Constructive, where the experimental group received a significantly higher score than the control group. See Table 4.

Hypothesis 2: Affective/Cognitive

Hypothesis H_2: There will be no significant difference in gain between subjects in the RR and NRR groups in terms of the feeling level of their responses to clients.

Table 5 presents a summary of the results of applying "t" tests of significance to the facilitative responses of the subjects as measured on the Counselor Verbal Response Scale. The nonfacilitative components of these four dichotomized dimensions are not shown in Table 5 since we are focusing on possible gains in facilitative responses and a gain in one component of a dimension is necessarily accompanied by an equal loss in the score of the other component, and vice versa.

Since Table 5 shows that there was no significant difference in the posttest scores of the control and experimental groups, this hypothesis is accepted.

Hypothesis H_{2A}: There will be no significant gain in feeling level of the responses to their clients for subjects in the RR group.

Table 4
Analysis of Pretest POI Scores
Control vs Experimental Groups

POI symbol**	Control mean	S.D.	Experimental mean	S.D.	Mean difference	U*	Significance
Ti	7.88	3.13	6.21	2.77	-1.67	34.5	NS
Tc	15.13	3.13	16.80	2.77	1.67	34.5	NS
O	43.75	6.99	39.94	9.60	-3.81	50.5	NS
I	78.00	8.03	85.43	9.55	7.43	34.5	NS
SAV	18.75	3.88	20.51	2.79	1.76	43.5	NS
Ex	17.75	4.31	20.79	3.71	3.04	39	NS
Fr	15.63	1.37	16.86	2.72	1.23	32	NS
S	12.38	1.64	13.79	1.67	1.41	34.5	NS
Sr	11.50	2.28	11.87	2.21	0.37	55.5	NS
Sa	14.13	3.01	14.79	2.72	0.66	48.5	NS
Nc	8.75	2.32	12.29	1.54	3.54	14	p<.05 Cont.>Exp.
Sy	6.50	.83	6.86	1.09	0.36	48	NS
A	15.88	1.26	15.87	2.73	- .01	49.5	NS
C	17.88	2.56	19.16	2.42	1.28	43	NS

*Mann-Whitney U.
**See Figure 1 for symbol description.

Table 5
Analysis of CVRS* Scores for Facilitative Responses

Facilitative Response**	"t" Score	Significance
Dimension: Affective		
Control: Pretest vs. Posttest	1.208	NS
Exper.: Pretest vs. Posttest	1.466	NS
Cont. vs. Exper.: Pretest	0.383	NS
Cont. vs. Exper.: Posttest	1.566	NS
Dimension: Understanding		
Control: Pretest vs. Posttest	1.325	NS
Exper.: Pretest vs. Posttest	2.790	p<.05 Post>Pre
Cont. vs. Exper.: Pretest	1.748	NS
Cont. vs. Exper.: Posttest	2.511	p<.05 Exp.>Cont.
Dimension: Specific		
Control: Pretest vs. Posttest	0.504	NS
Exper.: Pretest vs. Posttest	1.833	NS
Cont. vs. Exper.: Pretest	1.011	NS
Cont. vs. Exper.: Posttest	1.226	NS
Dimension: Exploratory		
Control: Pretest vs. Posttest	1.678	NS
Exper.: Pretest vs. Posttest	0.766	NS
Cont. vs. Exper.: Pretest	0.994	NS
Cont. vs. Exper.: Posttest	1.175	NS

*Counselor Verbal Response Scale.
**Facilitative responses only are analyzed since scores are in terms of proportion of responses.

No significant gain was found between the pretest and posttest scores of the RR group; therefore this hypothesis is accepted. See Table 5.

Hypothesis H_{2B}: There will be no significant gain in feeling level in the responses to their clients for subjects in the NRR group.

Since no significant gain was found, Table 5, between the pretest and posttest scores of the NRR group, this hypothesis is accepted.

Hypothesis 3: Understanding/Nonunderstanding

Hypothesis H_3: There will be no significant difference in gain in understanding of client responses between subjects in the RR and the NRR groups.

As shown in Table 5, a significant difference ($p<.05$) was found in gain in understanding between the posttest scores of the experimental group compared with the control group. Therefore, this hypothesis is rejected.

Hypothesis H_{3A}: There will be no significant difference in gain in understanding of client responses for subjects in the RR group.

Table 5 reflects the finding of a significant gain in understanding in the posttest scores of the RR group compared with their pretest scores. Therefore, this hypothesis is rejected.

Hypothesis H$_{3B}$: There will be no significant gain in understanding of client responses for subjects in the NRR group.

No significant gain was found between the posttest and pretest scores of the NRR group, as indicated in Table 5. Therefore, this hypothesis is accepted.

Hypothesis 4: Specific/Nonspecific

Hypothesis H$_4$: There will be no difference in gain between the RR and the NRR groups in the degree of specificity of responses to their clients.

Application of the "t" test of significance to the posttest scores of the two groups found the differences not significant at the 95 percent level of confidence. This hypothesis, therefore, is accepted.

Hypothesis H$_{4A}$: There will be no significant gain in the degree of specificity of responses to clients for subjects in the RR group.

No significant gain was found between the pretest and posttest scores of the RR group and, therefore, this hypothesis is accepted.

Hypothesis H$_{4B}$: There will be no significant gain in the degree of specificity of responses to clients for subjects in the NRR group.

No significant gain was found between the pretest and posttest scores of the NRR group, as indicated in Table 5. Hypothesis H$_{4B}$, therefore, is accepted.

Hypothesis 5: Exploratory/Nonexploratory

Hypothesis H_5: There will be no significant difference in gain between subjects in the RR and the NRR groups in ability to give responses that lead clients to further self-exploration.

The difference in the posttest scores of the two groups were not significant ($p < .05$) and this hypothesis is accepted.

Hypothesis H_{5A}: There will be no significant gain in ability to give responses that lead clients to further self-exploration for subjects in the RR group.

No significant differences were found in the pretest and posttest scores of the subjects in the RR group. This hypothesis, therefore, is accepted.

Hypothesis H_{5B}: There will be no significant gain in ability to give responses that lead clients to further self-exploration for subjects in the NRR group.

The pretest and posttest scores of subjects in the NRR group revealed no significant gain. Hypothesis H_{5B} is accepted for that reason.

The analysis of our results thus far indicates that, although the RR group scored significant gains in a broad range of self-actualizing values, which replicates some of the results reported in Chapter II (Seeman, Nidich, & Banta, 1972), these gains were translated into higher ratios of facilitiative responses only in the dimension of understanding.

The RR group gained in this dimension both in relation to its own pretest score and vis-a-vis the control group in the posttest scores. However, when we examine the actual group means which are shown in Table 6 and Table 7 in terms of actual proportions (percentages) of responses, a somewhat different picture emerges. Table 6 shows that whereas the control group actually decreased their proportion of facilitative responses for each of the four dimensions, the experimental group showed an increase in every case. This group's affective, understanding and specific responses increased by 50 percent or more while its exploratory responses increased by almost 18 percent, comparing posttest to pretest scores. If we sum the group means of just the facilitative responses for each dimension we find that the combined group mean proportion went from 46.8 percent down to 37.9 percent for the control group while increasing from 35.8 percent to 51.4 percent for the experimental group.

A comparison of the pretest scores of the two groups, as shown in Table 7, reveals that the average proportion of all facilitative responses of the experimental group was 11 points, or almost 31 percent lower than that for the control group. By the time of the posttest, however, the experimental group had a combined mean proportion that was 13.5 points and 26 percent higher than the control subjects. These are impressive gains by the experimental group but not large enough, except in the case of the understanding

Table 6
Comparisons of Group Mean Facilitative Responses
RR* & NRR** Groups: Pretest vs Posttest

Dimensions	Mean Proportion		Point Difference	Percent Change
	Pretest	Posttest		
RR (Experimental) Group				
Affective	15.3	28.4	+13.1	+85.6
Cognitive	84.7	71.6	-13.1	-15.5
Understanding	55.1	82.4	+27.3	+49.5
Nonunderstanding	44.9	17.6	-27.3	-60.0
Specific	27.8	41.9	+14.1	+50.7
Nonspecific	72.2	58.1	-14.1	-19.5
Exploratory	44.9	52.8	+7.9	+17.6
Nonexploratory	55.1	47.2	-7.9	-14.3
Mean Proportion of All Facilitative Res.	35.8	51.4	+15.6	+43.6
NRR (Control) Group				
Affective	17.9	12.1	-5.8	-32.4
Cognitive	82.1	87.9	+5.8	+7.1
Understanding	75.9	65.1	-10.8	-44.8
Nonunderstanding	24.1	34.9	+10.8	+44.8
Exploratory	55.6	41.5	-14.1	-25.4
Nonexploratory	44.4	58.5	+14.1	+31.8
Mean Proportion of All Facilitative Res.	46.8	37.9	-8.9	-19.0

*RR: Relaxation Response (Experimental Group).
**NRR: Non-Relaxation Response (Control Group).

59

Table 7
Comparison of Group Mean Facilitative Responses
Pretest and Posttest Scores: RR* vs NRR**

| Dimensions | Mean Proportion | | Point Difference | Percent Change |
	RR	NRR		
Pretest Responses				
Affective	15.3	17.9	-2.6	-17.0
Cognitive	84.7	82.1	+2.6	+3.1
Understanding	55.1	75.9	-20.8	-37.7
Nonunderstanding	44.9	24.1	-20.8	+46.3
Specific	27.8	37.9	-10.1	-36.3
Nonspecific	72.2	62.1	+10.1	+14.0
Exploratory	44.9	55.6	-10.7	-23.8
Nonexploratory	55.1	44.4	+10.7	+19.4
Mean Proportion of All Facilitative Res.	35.8	46.8	-11.0	-30.7
Posttest Responses				
Affective	28.4	12.1	+16.3	+57.4
Cognitive	71.6	87.9	-16.3	-22.8
Understanding	82.4	65.1	+17.3	+21.0
Nonunderstanding	17.6	34.9	-17.3	-98.3
Specific	41.9	32.8	+9.1	+21.7
Nonspecific	58.1	67.2	-9.1	-15.7
Exploratory	52.8	41.5	+11.3	+21.4
Nonexploratory	47.2	58.5	-11.3	-23.9
Mean Proportion of All Facilitative Res.	51.4	37.9	+13.5	+26.3

*RR: Relaxation Response (Experimental Group).
**NRR: Non-Relaxation Response (Control Group).

dimension, to conclude according to the "t" statistic test, that such differences could be expected in only 5 percent of the cases in samples drawn from the same population.

But this result stems from examining each of our hypotheses, and therefore, each dimension separately from the other. If we apply our "t" test statistic to the average proportion of all facilitative responses combined, as shown in Tables 6 and 7 ("Mean Proportion of All Facilitative Responses"), we get another perspective of the results.

Table 8 shows the results of applying "t" tests of significance at the 95 percent confidence level ($p < .05$) to the mean proportion of all four facilitative dimension responses combined. These results show a significant difference between the pretest and posttest scores of the control group which reflects the decrease in proportion of facilitative responses pointed out above. On the other hand, the experimental group showed significant gains both in their own posttest scores compared to pretest, and in their posttest scores compared to those of the control group.

Our conclusion, then, is that when individual dimensions are considered, the experimental group shows gains at the level of confidence we chose to employ, only in the dimension of understanding. But there was a sufficient gain in each dimension to produce an overall significant gain when all facilitative responses in all dimensions are considered as a whole. No significant difference was found between the pretest scores of the two groups.

As stated above, the nonparametric Mann-Whitney U and the Wilcoxon Signed-Rank Statistic were used to test measures of self-actualization in the POI and to serve as a criterion for accepting or rejecting hypothesis 1. For comparison purposes, the parametric "t" statistic was also used to test the measures of Self-Actualization in hypothesis 1. The results of these tests of significance are given for information in Appendix E.

Table 11 of Appendix E agrees with Table 1 in the text in the analysis of posttest POI scores, control vs experimental, except that the "t" statistic found a significant gain in Self-Regard (Sr) while the Mann-Whitney U did not. On the other hand, the Mann-Whitney U indicates a significant gain in the Acceptance of Aggression while the "t" test statistic does not. In all important respects, however, both tests tend to corroborate the findings of this study.

Table 9 tabulates the number of responses by each counselor in the 10 minute segment of tapes which was used in rating counselor responses. These figures indicate that there was no significant variation in the counselor response level between groups or between tests of the same group. Therefore, counselor response level is not considered to be a contributing factor to any variations in results between treatment groups.

Table 8
Analysis of Mean Group Proportions
All Facilitative Responses on CVRS

Treatment Group	"t" Statistic	Significance
Control: Posttest vs Pretest	4.19	p<.05 Pre>Post
Experimental: Posttest vs Pretest	3.77	p<.05 Post>Pre
Pretest: Exp. vs Control	2.96	NS
Posttest: Exp. vs Control	6.86	p<.05 Exp.>Cont.

Table 9
Counselor Response Level

Subject Number	Control Group		Experimental Group	
	Pretest	Posttest	Pretest	Posttest
1	19	9	19	16
2	23	12	26	34
3	12	22	24	18
4	23	23	20	14
5	16	14	13	20
6	10	15	12	6
7	10	18	24	7
8	9	17	17	17
9			9	11
10			14	18
11			19	15
12			16	14
Total Responses	122	130	222	190
Average Number	15.25	16.25	18.50	15.80

The average number of times per week that each subject in the experimental group practiced Relaxation Response is tabulated in Table 10. These data were computed from the calendars maintained by each of the 12 subjects whose CVRS responses have been tabulated in this report. As can be seen in the figures, there was considerable variation as to the number of times the members of the experimental group practiced meditation. The bottom quartile averaged only 4.8 meditation sessions for the 10 week period while the top quartile averaged 11 sessions. The overall average was 7.1 practice sessions per week, however, all quartiles but the top one averaged less than the group average. No attempt was made to collate calendar information with test scores since the test results were not identified by subject name. Therefore, no correlation between amount of meditation and gains in facilitative response dimensions could be carried out.

Table 10
Average Number of Relaxation Response Sessions
Per Week by Members of Experimental Group

Subject No.	Quartile No.	Av. No. Weekly RR Sessions	Quartile Average
1	1	4.2	4.8
2		4.8	
3		5.5	
4	2	5.6	5.9
5		6.1	
6		6.1	
7	3	6.4	6.7
8		6.8	
9		7.0	
10	4	7.6	11.0
11		12.1	
12		13.2	
Group Average		7.1	
Group Median		6.2	

Table 11
Scoring Categories for the Personal
Orientation Inventory

Number of Items	Scale Number	Symbol	Description	Number of Items	Scale Number	Symbol	Description
I. Ratio Scores				26	10	Sa	SELF-ACCEPTANCE Measures affirmation or acceptance of self in spite of weaknesses or deficiencies
23	1/2	T_I/T_C	TIME RATIO Time Incompetence/ Time Competence – measures degree to which one is "present" oriented				
127	3/4	O/I	SUPPORT RATIO Other/Inner – measures whether reactivity orientation is basically toward others or self	16	11	Nc	NATURE OF MAN Measures degree of the constructive view of the nature of man, masculinity, feminity
II. Sub-Scales				9	12	Sy	SYNERGY Measures ability to be synergistic, to transcend dichotomies
26	5	SAV	SELF-ACTUALIZING VALUE Measures affirmation of primary values of self-actualizing persons				
32	6	Ex	EXISTENTIALITY Measures ability to situationally or existentially react without rigid adherence to principles	25	13	A	ACCEPTANCE OF AGGRESSION Measures ability to accept one's natural aggressiveness as opposed to defensiveness, denial, and repression of aggression
23	7	Fr	FEELING REACTIVITY Measures sensitivity of responsiveness to one's own needs and feelings	28	14	C	CAPACITY FOR INTIMATE CONTACT Measures ability to develop contactful intimate relationships with other human beings, unencumbered by expectations and obligations
18	8	S	SPONTANEITY Measures freedom to react spontaneously or to be oneself				
16	9	Se	SELF-REGARD Measures affirmation of self because of worth or strength				

CHAPTER V

SUMMARY, CONCLUSIONS AND IMPLICATIONS

Summary

This study was designed to measure the effects of a meditation technique upon the behavior of a group of para-professionals acting as counselors. Of primary interest was the question of whether or not a meditation technique developed by Benson and referred to as the Relaxation Response resulted in the enhancement of the positive personality characteristics which have been correlated with counselor effectiveness. It has been found (Carkhuff, 1969b, pp. 84-90) that the degree to which the helping person offers high levels of empathy, warmth, respect, concreteness and genuineness is related directly to client growth. Available research on meditation suggests that these are the very qualities which have been found to be enhanced by meditation. Previous research (see page 21, above, for examples) found that meditators scored significantly higher than nonmeditators on such scales as inner directedness, time competence, self-actualization values, spontaneity and self-acceptance. These are among the qualities measured by

66

the Personal Orientation Inventory (POI) (Shostrom, 1966), one of the research instruments used in this study.

The specific behavior examined in this study was the counselor's responses to client communications in terms of four dichotomized dimensions measured by the Counselor Verbal Response Scale (CVRS) (Kagan & Krathwohl, 1967), which is the other principal research instrument used in this study. The four dichotomized dimensions included in the CVRS are: 1) affective/cognitive; 2) understanding/nonunderstanding; 3) specific/nonspecific; and 4) exploratory/nonexploratory. Counselor response in a client-counselor interaction was rated on each of the four dimensions of the rating scale, with each interaction being judged as an independent unit. The counselor's responses were judged primarily on the manner in which he responded to the verbal elements of the client's communication. The judges rated each counselor response to the client on each of the dimensions of the scale. Totals were tallied after responses had been dichotomized on each dimension on two five minute segments of each tape.

The study population consisted of 22 paraprofessional counselor-candidates who were attending their first term at the Santa Fe Community College Human Services Department. These subjects were randomly assigned to one of two groups-- an eight member control group and a 14 member experimental group. Two of the tapes for the experimental group subjects

were lost and our CVRS analysis, therefore, was based upon
12 experimental group members, while the POI analysis covers
all 14 experimental group members.

The members of each group were pretested with the
Personal Orientation Inventory, an essentially self-
administered instrument developed by Shostrom (1964, 1966).
The POI consists of 150 two-choice paired opposite statements of personal values which are believed to be important
in the development of positive mental health. Scores are
reported on two major scales and 10 secondary scales as out-
lined on page 34, above.

After completing the initial POI each subject, acting
as counselor, taped an interview with a fellow student,
acting as client. Subjects in the experimental group then
received instructions in the meditation technique developed
by Benson, called the Relaxation Response. They were given
forms on which to record the number of times and the time
of day that they practiced meditation during the ensuing 10
weeks in a regular daily program of meditation which they
were asked to undertake. Members of the control group were
told that they would receive instruction in RR at the end
of the semester.

At the end of 10 weeks all the subjects were given the
POI for the second time and were given a second cassette
tape on which to record a posttest counseling tape.

Four graduate students in counseling psychology were selected as raters for the two sets of counseling tapes. They were trained as raters by a counseling psychologist. Ten minute segments of each tape were rated by each of two raters. In scoring the CVRS the ratings of the two raters were averaged.

Results

Significant gains by the experimental group compared to the control group were found in 5 of the 12 scales of the POI. The experimental group evidenced gains compared with the control group in Inner Directedness, Existentiality, Spontaneity, Self-Acceptance and Acceptance of Aggressive Tendencies in Oneself. On the other hand, the control group posttest scores showed a significant ($p < .05$) gain in Other Directedness, a nonself-actualizing factor, relative to the posttest scores of the experimental group.

All of these gains were found to be significant by use of the Mann-Whitney U (see Table 1). Also, all of these gains were corroborated as significant ($p < .05$) by the "t" statistic, with the exception of Acceptance of Aggression. In addition, the "t" statistic indicated a significant gain in Self-Regard.

Use of the Wilcoxon Signed-Rank Statistic validated significant gains in the experimental group's posttest scores compared with those of the pretest in the following dimensions: Inner Directedness, Spontaneity, Self-Regard and Self-Acceptance.

There was a significant difference between the pretest scores of the experimental versus the control group only in the dimension, Nature of Man, Constructive, with the experimental group ranking higher. The Wilcoxon Signed-Rank Statistic revealed no significant gains or losses in the posttest scores of the control group compared with its pretest scores.

Performance of "t" tests of significance on the pretest and posttest scores on the Counselor Verbal Response Scale of the two groups revealed no significant differences except in the understanding-nonunderstanding dimension. The RR group's posttest scores showed significant gains compared with their own pretest score and compared to the control group's posttest scores. The pretest scores of the two groups yielded no significant differences at all.

Thus there were no significant gains or losses in the other three dichotomized dimensions: affective/cognitive; specific/nonspecific; and exploratory/nonexploratory. However, comparisons of the actual group proportions expressed in percentage terms reveals impressive percentage gains in the posttest scores of the experimental group compared to their pretest figures and compared to the posttest scores of the control group. Whereas these gains were not great enough by individual dimension to rule out the possibility

that they could have occurred in a similar pretest sample
drawn from the same population, when the proportions for
all dimensions were averaged for facilitative responses only,
significant differences did become apparent. Applying the
"t" test to the mean proportion of all facilitative responses
from all dimensions for each group revealed that: the
control group registered significant losses in the proportion
of facilitative responses; the experimental group exhibited
significant gains in the overall proportion of facilitative
responses, posttest versus pretest; and that the experimental group gained significantly in their proportion of
facilitative responses vis-a-vis the control group, based
upon a comparison of their posttest scores.

Conclusions

In this study we attempted to measure the affects, if
any, on counselor behavior of a meditation technique,
Relaxation Response, which was developed by Benson. The
research design called for measuring in an experimental
group any gains in self-actualization that might be
attributable to meditation and the Relaxation Response.
Since the control group was chosen from the same population
as the experimental group and all other conditions and
influences were assumed to be equal--for example, the training that both groups were receiving at the Human Services
Department--any significant gains by the experimental group

might be attributed to the program of meditation carried out by the members of that group.

The POI scores indicated that significant gains in a broad spectrum of self-actualizing values were made by the RR group. Particularly important was the gain by the RR group in Inner Directedness, one of the two principal scales of the POI. Inner, or self-directed individuals are guided primarily by internal principles and motivations, one of the attributes of positive mental health.

Did this gain by the experimental group in self-actualizing values translate itself into more effective counseling behavior as measured by the CVRS? Significant gains in desirable counselor behavior were found only in the dimension of understanding. No significant gains were noted in the facilitative responses characterized as affective, specific and exploratory. A possible explanation for this result may be found in distinguishing between the characterizations of counselor response in the CVRS model. The habit of responding to client verbalizations in specific terms or in terms that encourage further exploration could be thought of as depending on learned technique rather than on basic personality factors. In contrast, the quality of understanding, particularly in the context of the interactions between a counselor and client, would seem to depend more on the stage of personality development and experience than on specific techniques that can be taught in a classroom situation.

If this premise is accepted, then it would seem logical that new gains in a person's level of self-actualization and in basic positive personality characteristics would first manifest themselves in a greater capacity to understand the communications of another human being. As we saw on page 3 above, Rogers (1957), in describing the necessary characteristics of effective counselors, linked "empathic understanding of the client" and the "self-congruence of the counselor." Thus in our present study, we may conclude that the measured gains in self-actualization were linked at the basic personality level to gains in the capacity for understanding. We may also conclude that such gains at the level of personality development may not be translated immediately into specific professional skills or techniques (a verbal bag of tools) which require learning. This would appear to be especially true of the subjects of this study who were students in the initial stages of learning their profession.

Our principal conclusion, based upon the results of this study, is that the Benson Relaxation Response technique of meditation appears to offer one means of acquiring and developing the positive personality characteristics which have been linked to effective counseling. The first results of such a meditation technique may manifest themselves in a capacity for increased understanding of another's communication.

Limitations of the Study

Generalization based on this study are limited to the Santa Fe Community College Human Services Program for paraprofessional counselors. The sampling procedures did not make allowance for generalizing outside of this population. A small sample size of twenty-two further limits generalizability.

The amount of time in which subjects engaged in the practice of the Relaxation Response (RR) is an important factor. The overall length of time that the experimental group practiced the RR was 10 weeks. The average number of times per week was 7 times. However, there was a wide variance in the meditation schedules of the individual members, see Table 10. All quartiles except the top quartile had a practice rate of less than the group average of 7 times a week. It may be that a more consistent schedule may produce more definite results. (See Implications for Future Research #5).

Implications for Future Research

The findings of this investigation suggest that a meditation procedure, namely the Relaxation Response (RR), can be adopted by a paraprofessional counseling program. Research cited in this study demonstrated the importance of positive personality characteristics as it relates to counselor

75

effectiveness. The present study also suggests training designed to aid in the development of self-actualizing attributes in counselors. This type of training may be considered as important to counselors as the formal training in mechanical skills and theory.

The following suggestions may be of value to those interested in further research on this subject.

1) To further investigate the quality of meditation being practiced by each student. Researchers can carefully monitor not only the actual amount of time spent in the RR, but the quality of the experience by means of biofeedback equipment. Biofeedback equipment which measures brain waves (EEG), muscle tension (EMG), or galvanic skin resistance (GSR) may contribute to further exploration and development of student potentials.

2) A longitudinal design could be used to investigate the long term effect of the RR on the personality characteristics of paraprofessional counselors. Also, this type of design could allow more time for students to translate their personal perceptions from the RR experience to behaviors measurable by the research instruments. Further research is needed to explore the relationship of time spent in meditation and personal growth.

3) The present study indicates the need for further investigation of the correlation of the affective content of counselor responses with the degree of self-actualization of the counselor. We have attempted to explain the fact that the specific and exploratory dimensions of the CVRS did not increase in tandem with the gains in measures of self-actualization with the assumption that these dimensions are more dependent upon skill-training than on the development of positive personality traits. However, a person gaining in self-actualizing values would, by our definition, also be increasing his capacity for empathy and there-fore, would be expected to manifest this empathy by increased levels of feeling content versus cognitive content in his responses to clients. The reason for the failure of our experimental group to show significant gains in the proportion of these responses needs further study.

4) Researchers may further investigate the interaction effects of self-actualization, meditation, and counselor effectiveness. For example, one question not answered by the present research is, do initially high self-actualized individuals show significantly greater gains from practice of the RR than initially low self-actualized individuals? More research is necessary to answer this question.

5) As mentioned in the Limitations of the Study, the amount of time spent in the practice of the RR was shown to be highly variable. Future research may show that a more consistent schedule of meditation can produce more definite results. Therefore, researchers may wish to incorporate into their experimental design methods to insure a minimum period of time in which the subjects engage in practice of the RR. For example, incentives such as the payment of fees to subjects may be advantageous, however, more research is needed to verify this conclusion.

6) In the counseling relationship, clients respond to both the verbal and nonverbal behaviors of the counselor. In addition to verbal communication, the counselor uses facial, postural and gestural modes of communication. Therefore, future research may be supplemented by videotape recordings of the client/counselor interaction to observe changes in both verbal and nonverbal communications as a result of the RR training.

Continued research is needed which focuses directly upon the kinds of experience which will facilitate the counselor's personal awareness, integration and psychological maturity.

APPENDIX A

How to Bring Forth the Relaxation Response

and

Eliciting the Relaxation Response

How to Bring Forth the Relaxation Response

(1) A Quiet Environment.

Ideally, you should choose a quiet, calm environment with as few distractions as possible. A quiet room is suitable, as is a place of worship. The quiet environment contributes to the effectiveness of the repeated work or phrase by making it easier to eliminate distracting thoughts.

(2) A Mental Device.

To shift the mind from logical, externally oriented thought, there should be a constant stimulus: a sound, word, or phrase repeated silently or aloud; or fixed gazing at an object. Since one of the major difficulties in the elicitation of the Relaxation Response is "mind wandering," the repetition of the word or phrase is a way to help break the train of distracting thoughts. Your eyes are usually closed if you are using a repeated sound or word; of course, your eyes are open if you are gazing. Attention to the normal rhythm of breathing is also useful and enhances the repetition of the sound or the word.

(3) A Passive Attitude.

When distracting thoughts occur, they are to be dis-regarded and attention redirected to the repetition or

gazing; you should not worry about how well you are performing the technique, because this may well prevent the
Relaxation Response from occurring. Adopt a "let it happen"
attitude. The passive attitude is perhaps the most important element in eliciting the Relaxation Response. Distracting thoughts will occur. Do not worry about them.
When these thoughts do present themselves and you become
aware of them, simply return to the repetition of the mental
device. These other thoughts do not mean you are performing
the technique incorrectly. They are to be expected.

(4) A Comfortable Position.

A comfortable posture is important so that there is no
undue muscular tension. Some methods call for a sitting
position. A few practitioners use the cross-legged "lotus"
position of the Yogi. If you are lying down, there is a
tendency to fall asleep. As we have noted previously, the
various postures of kneeling, swaying, or sitting in cross-
legged position are believed to have evolved to prevent
falling asleep. You should be comfortable and relaxed.

Eliciting the Relaxation Response

(1) In a quiet environment, sit in a comfortable position.
(2) Close your eyes.
(3) Deeply relax your muscles, beginning at your feet and
     progressing up to your face--feet, calves, thighs, lower
     torso, chest, shoulders, neck, head. Allow them to
     remain deeply relaxed.

(4)   Breathe through your nose. Become aware of your
       breathing. As you breathe in, say the sound "So"
       silently to yourself and as you breathe out say "Hum."
       Thus: breathe in--"So" . . . breathe out with "Hum."
       In, "So" and out with "Hum." . . .

(5)   Continue this practice for twenty minutes. You may
       open your eyes to check the time, but do not use an
       alarm. When you finish, sit quietly for several
       minutes, at first with your eyes closed and later with
       your eyes open.

(6)   Remember not to worry about whether you are successful
       in achieving a deep level of relaxation--maintain a
       passive attitude and permit relaxation to occur at its
       own pace. When distracting thoughts occur, ignore
       them and continue to repeat "So-Hum" as you breathe.
       The technique should be practiced twice daily, and not
       within two hours after any meal, since the digestive
       processes seem to interfere with the elicitation of
       the expected.

APPENDIX B

Counselor Verbal Response Scale

Counselor Verbal Response Scale Rating Sheet

Counselor Verbal Response Scale

Description of Rating Dimensions

I. Affective-cognitive dimension

The affective-cognitive dimension indicates whether a counselor's response refers to any affective component of a client's communication or concerns itself primarily with the cognitive component of that communication.

A. Affective responses: Affective responses generally make reference to emotions, feelings, fears, etc. The judge's rating is solely by the content and/or intent of the counselor's response, regardless of whether it be reflection, clarification or interpretation. These responses attempt to maintain the focus on the affective component of a client's communication. Thus they may:

(a) Refer directly to an explicit or implicit reference to affect (either verbal or nonverbal) on the part of the client.

(b) Encourage an expression of affect on the part of the client. Example: "How does it make you feel when your parents argue?"

(c) Approve of an expression of affect on the part of the client. Example: "It doesn't hurt to

83

let your feelings out once in a while, does it?"

(d)   Presents a model for the use of affect by the client.   Example: "If somebody treated me like that, I'd really be mad."

Special care must be taken in rating responses which use the word "feel."   For example, in the statement "do you feel that your student teaching experience is helping you get the idea of teaching?" the phrase "do you feel that" really means "do you think that."   Similarly, the expression "How are you feeling?" is often used in a matter-of-fact, conversation manner.   Thus, although the verb "to feel" is used in both these examples, these statements do not represent responses which would be judged "affective."

B.   Cognitive Responses: Cognitive responses deal primarily with the cognitive element of a client's communication.   Frequently, such responses seek information of factual nature.   They generally maintain the interaction on the cognitive level.   Such responses may:

(a)   Refer directly to the cognitive component of the client's statement.

Example: "So then you're thinking about switching your major to chemistry?"

(b)   Seeks further information of a factual nature from the client.

Example: "What were your grades last term?"

      (c)   Encourage the client to continue to respond
at the cognitive level.

          Example: "How did you get interested in art?"

II. Understanding-nonunderstanding dimension

The understanding-nonunderstanding dimension indicates whether a counselor's response communicates to the client that the counselor understands or is seeking to understand the client's basic communication. This encourages the client to continue to gain insight into the nature of his concerns.

A. Understanding responses: Understanding responses communicate to the client that the counselor understands the client's communication--the counselor makes appropriate reference to what the client is expressing or trying to express both verbally and nonverbally--or the counselor is clearly seeking enough information of either a cognitive or affective nature to gain such understanding. Such responses:

      (a)   Directly communicate an understanding of the
client's communication.

          Example: "In other words, you really want to
be treated like a man."

      (b)   Seek further information from the client in
such a way as to facilitate both the counselors' and the clients' understanding of the
basic problems.

          Example: "What does being a man mean to you?"

      (c)   Reinforce or give approval or client communica-
tions which exhibit understanding.

Example: CL: "I guess then, when people
criticize me, I'm afraid they'll
leave me."

CO: "I see you're beginning to make
some connection between your
behavior and your feelings."

B. <u>Nonunderstanding responses</u>: Nonunderstanding
responses are those in which the counselor fails to understand the client's basic communication or makes no attempt
to obtain <u>appropriate</u> information from the client. In
essence, nonunderstanding implies misunderstanding. Such
responses:

(a) Communicate misunderstanding of the client's
basic concern.

Example: CL: "When he said that, I just
turned red and clenched my
fists."

CO: "Some people don't say nice
things."

(b) Seek information which may be irrelevant to
the client's communication.

Example: CL: "I seem to have a hard time
getting along with my brothers."

CO: "Do all your brothers live at
home with you?"

     (c)   Squelch client understanding or move the focus
to another irrelevant area.

       Example: CL: "I guess I'm really afraid that
                             other people will laugh at me."
                  CO: "We're the butt of other poeple's
                             jokes sometimes."
       Example: CL: "Sometimes I really hate my aunt."
                  CO: "Will things be better when you
                             go to college?"

III. Specific/nonspecific dimension

The specific-nonspecific dimension indicates whether
the counselor's response delineates the client's problems
and is central to the client's communication or whether the
response does not specify the client's concern. In essence,
it describes whether the counselor deals with client's
communication in a general, vague, or peripheral manner, or
"zeros in" on the core of the client's communication. NB:
A response judged to be nonunderstanding must also be nonspecific since it would, by definition, misunderstand the
client's communication and not help the client to delineate
his concerns. Responses judged understanding might be
either specific (core) or nonspecific (peripheral) i.e.,
they would be peripheral if the counselor conveys only a
vague idea that a problem exists or "flirts" with the idea
rather than helping the client delineate some of the dimensions of his concerns.

A. Specific responses: Specific responses focus on
the core concerns being presented either explicitly or
implicitly, verbally or nonverbally, by the client. Such
responses:

(a) Delineate more closely the client's basic
concerns.

Example: "This vague feeling you have when
you get in tense situations--is it
anger or fear?"

(b) Encourage the client to discriminate among
stimuli affecting him.

Example: "Do you feel _____ in all your
classes or in only some classrooms?"

(c) Reward the client for being specific.

Example: CL: "I guess I feel this way most
often with someone who reminds
me of my father."

CO: "So as you put what others say
in perspective the whole world
doesn't seem so bad; it's only
when someone you value, like
Father, doesn't pay any attention
that you feel hurt."

B. Nonspecific responses: Nonspecific responses indicate that the counselor is not focusing on the basic concerns of the client or is not yet able to help the client

differentiate among various stimuli. Such responses either
miss the problem area completely (such responses are also
nonunderstanding) or occur when the counselor is seeking to
understand the client's communication and has been presented
with only vague bits of information about the client's
concern. Thus, such responses:

(a) Fail to delineate the client's concern and
cannot bring them into sharper focus.

Example: "It seems your problem isn't very
clear--can you tell me more about it?"

(b) Completely miss the basic concerns being presented by the client even though the counselor
may ask for specific details.

Example: CL: "I've gotten all A's this year
and I still feel lousy."

CO: "What were your grades before
then?"

(c) Discourage the client from bringing his concerns
into sharper focus.

Example: "You and your sister argue all the
time. What do other people think of
your sister?"

IV. Exploratory-nonexploratory

The exploratory-nonexploratory dimension indicates
whether a counselor's response permits or encourages the
client to explore his cognitive or affective concerns, or

whether the response limits a client's exploration of these concerns.

A. <u>Exploratory responses</u>: Exploratory responses encourage and permit the client latitude and involvement in his response. They may focus on relevant aspects of the client's affective or cognitive concerns but clearly attempt to encourage further exploration by the client. Such responses are often open-ended and/or are delivered in a manner permitting the client freedom and flexibility in response. These responses:

(a) Encourage the client to explore his own concerns.

Example: Cognitive--"You're not sure what you want to major in, is that it?"

Affective--"Maybe some of these times you're getting mad at yourself, what do you think?"

(b) Assist the client to explore by providing him with possible alternatives designed to increase his range of responses.

Example: Cognitive--"What are some of the other alternatives that you have to history as a major?"

Affective--"In these situations, do you feel angry, mad, helpless, or what?"

(c) Reward the client for exploratory behavior.

Example: Cognitive--"It seems that you've considered a number of alternatives for a major, that's good."

Affective--"So you're beginning to wonder if you always want to be treated like a man."

B. Nonexploratory responses: Nonexploratory responses either indicate no understanding of the client's basic communication, or so structure and limit the client's responses that they inhibit the exploratory process. The responses give the client little opportunity to explore, expand, or express himself freely. Such responses:

Discourage further exploration on the part of the client.

Example: Cognitive--"You really resent your parents treating you like a child."

V. Effective-noneffective dimension

Ratings on the effective-noneffective dimension may be made independently of ratings on the other four dimensions of the scale. This rating is based solely upon the judge's professional impression of the appropriateness of the counselor's responses, that is, how adequately does the counselor's response deal with the client's verbal and nonverbal communication. This rating is not dependent on whether the response has been judged affective, cognitive, etc.

A rating of 4 indicates that the judge considers this response among the most appropriate possible. In the given situation, while a 3 indicates that the response is appropriate but not among the best. A rating of 2 indicates a neutral response which neither measurably affects client progress nor inhibits it, while a rating of 1 indicates a response which not only lacks basic understanding of the client's concerns but which in effect may be detrimental to the specified goals of client growth.

93

IPR COUNSELOR VERBAL RESPONSE RATING SCALE

Judge: _____   Subject: _____   Date: _____

DIMENSIONS

Responses	Affective	Cognitive	Understanding	Nonunderstanding	Specific	Nonspecific	Exploratory	Nonexploratory	Effective 4	Effective 3	Noneffective 2	Noneffective 1
1												
2												
3												
4												
5												
6												
7												
8												
9												
10												
11												
12												
13												
14												
15												
16												
17												
18												
19												
20												
21												
22												
23												
24												
25												
% of Responses												

Counselor Response Evaluation

TOTAL _____

TOTAL _____

APPENDIX C

Relaxation Response Calendar

To Help You Incorporate the Relax Response
In Your Daily Life, You May Use This Calendar

		Sun.	Mon.	Tues.	Wed.	Thurs.	Fri.	Sat.
Week 1	AM							
	PM							
Week 2	AM							
	PM							
Week 3	AM							
	PM							
Week 4	AM							
	PM							
Week 5	AM							
	PM							
Week 6	AM							
	PM							
Week 7	AM							
	PM							
Week 8	AM							
	PM							
Week 9	AM							
	PM							
Week 10	AM							
	PM							
Week 11	AM							
	PM							
Week 12	AM							
	PM							

Make a check mark ( ) in the appropriate place
each time you practice the Relaxation Response.

APPENDIX D

Demographic Data Sheet

HUMAN SERVICE TRAINING PROGRAM
Santa Fe Community College
August, 1976

Student Data Sheet

Please fill in the blanks or circle the answer that is
correct for you.

1. NAME: _____

    Local Area: _____

2. Race:

        A. white
        B. black
        C. other

3. Sex:

        A. male
        B. female

4. Age: _____

5. Marital Status (at present time):

        A. single (never married)
        B. married
        C. separated
        D. divorced
        E. widowed

6. Did you complete high school?

        A. yes
        B. no

7. Have you ever attended a college or junior college?

        A. yes
        B. no

8. Do you at present hold a college degree?

        A. yes
        B. no

9. If you hold a college degree, please indicate what type of degree.

    A. Associate of Arts (A.A.)
    B. Associate of Science (A.S.)
    C. Bachelor of Arts (B.A.)
    D. Bachelor of Science (B.S.)
    E. Other: _____

10. When you were growing up what was the job your father held most often? (Please be as specific as possible.)

    _____

11. If your mother worked while you were growing up, what was the job she held most often?

    _____

12. How many children do you have? _____

13. How many brothers do you have? _____

14. How many sisters do you have? _____

15. How many of these brothers and sisters are older than you? _____

16. In what city do you currently live? _____

17. How long have you lived there?

    A. less than 1 year
    B. 1 - 2 years
    C. 2 - 3 years
    D. 3 - 4 years
    E. 4 - 5 years
    F. longer than 5 years

18. How many different cities have you lived in during the last 5 years? _____

19. Did your father graduate from high school?

    A. yes
    B. no
    C. don't know

20. Did your father ever attend college?

    A. yes
    B. no
    C. don't know

21. Did your mother graduate from high school?

     A. yes
     B. no
     C. don't know

22. Did your mother ever attend college?

     A. yes
     B. no
     C. don't know

23. Which of the following reasons most influenced your decision to enroll in this program? (Please choose only one)

     A. Better job security
     B. To improve counseling skills
     C. Available training money
     D. Other: _____

Comments:

24. Previous work experience (start with most recent):

EMPLOYER	DATES	TYPE OF WORK
1. _____	_____	_____
2. _____	_____	_____
3. _____	_____	_____
4. _____	_____	_____

APPENDIX E

Additional Analyses of POI Scores

Table 12
Analysis of Posttest POI Scores
Control vs Experimental Groups

POI symbol**	"t" Statistic*	Significance
Tc		
I	2.26	p<.05 Exp.>Cont.
SAV		
Ex	2.12	p<.05 Exp.>Cont.
Fr		
S	2.27	p<.05 Exp.>Cont.
Sr	2.51	p<.05 Exp.>Cont.
Sa	3.03	p<.05 Exp.>Cont.
Nc		
Sy		
A		
C		

*Parametric "t" Statistic.
**See Figure 1 for symbol description.

Table 13
Analysis of Control Groups
Pretest vs Posttest POI Scores

POI symbol**	"t" Statistic*	Significance
Tc	Identical Means	NS
I	.266	NS
SAV	.738	NS
Ex	.173	NS
Fr	.107	NS
S	Identical Means	NS
Sr	.298	NS
Sa	.254	NS
Nc	1.850	NS
Sy	.523	NS
A	1.31	NS
C	.259	NS

*Parametric "t" Statistic.
**See Figure 1 for symbol description.

Table 14
Analysis of Experimental Group
Pretest vs Posttest POI Scores

POI symbol**	"t" Statistic	Significance
Tc	.182	NS
I	1.43	NS
SAV	.516	NS
Ex	.713	NS
Fr	.634	NS
S	1.36	NS
Sr	1.13	NS
Sa	2.68	$p<.05$ Post>Pre.
Nc	Identical Means	NS
Sy	.326	NS
A	.506	NS
C	.963	NS

*Parametric "t" Statistic.
**See Figure 1 for symbol description.

Table 15
Analysis of Pretest POI Scores
Control vs Experimental Groups

POI symbol**	"t" Statistic	Significance
Tc	1.44	NS
I	2.15	p<.05 Exp.>Cont.
SAV	1.32	NS
Ex	1.92	NS
Fr	1.45	NS
S	2.17	p<.05 Exp.>Cont.
Sr	.420	NS
Sa	.580	NS
Nc	4.57	p<.05 Exp.>Cont.
Sy	.940	NS
A	.120	NS
C	1.30	NS

*Parametric "t" Statistic.
**See Figure 1 for symbol description.

REFERENCES

Aspy, D. The relationship between the level of conditions offered by the teacher and academic achievement in third-grade pupils. Doctoral dissertation, University of Kentucky, 1965.

Beary, J.F. & Benson, H. A simple psychophysiologic technique which elicits the hypometabolic changes of the relaxation response. Psychosomatic Medicine, 1974, 36, 115-120.

Benson, H. The relaxation response. New York: William, Morrow and Co., Inc., 1975 (a).

Benson, H. The relaxation response. In M. Roman & C. Swencionis (Chair.), Biofeedback meditation and self-regulatory therapies. Symposium presented by the Dept. of Psychiatry, Albert Einstein College of Medicine, New York, Nov. 23, 1975 (b).

Benson, H., Alexander, S. & Feldman, C.L. Decreased premature ventricular contraction through use of the relaxation response in patients with stable ischaemic heart disease, Lancet, 1975, 793, (ii), 380-382.

Benson, H., Beary, J.F. & Carol, M.P. The relaxation response. Psychiatry, 1974, 37, 37-46.

Berenson, B. & Carkhuff, R. (Eds.) Sources of gain in counseling and psychotherapy. New York: Holt, Rinehart, and Winston, 1967.

Bergin, A.E. Some implications of psychotherapy research for therapeutic practice. Journal of Abnormal Psychology, 1966, 71, 235-246.

Bergin, A.E. & Solomon, S. Personality and performance correlates of emphathic understanding in psychotherapy. American Psychologist, 1963, 18, 393.

Bloomfield, H.H., Cain, M.P. & Jaffe, D.T. TM: Discovering inner energy and overcoming stress. New York: Delacorte, 1975.

106

Cannon, J.R. & Carkhuff, R.R. The effect of rater level
     of functioning and experience upon discrimination of
     facilitative conditions. Journal of Consulting
     Psychology, 1969, 33, 189-194.

Cannon, J.R. & Pierce, R.M. Order effects in the experi-
     mental manipulation of therapeutic conditions.
     Journal of Clinical Psychology, 1968, 24, 242-244.

Carkhuff, R.R. Counseling research, theory and practice.
     Journal of Counseling Psychology, 1966, 13, 467-480.

Carkhuff, R.R. Differential functioning of lay and pro-
     fessional helpers. Journal of Counseling Psychology,
     1968, 15, 117-126.

Carkhuff, R.R. Helping and human relations. Vol. 1.
     Selection and training. New York: Holt, Rinehart,
     and Winston, 1969 (a).

Carkhuff, R.R. Helping and human relations: A primer for
     lay and professional helpers. Vol. 2. Practice and
     research. New York: Holt, Rinehart, and Winston,
     1969 (b).

Carkhuff, R.R. The prediction of the effects of teacher
     counselor education: The development of communication
     and discrimination selection indexes. Counselor
     Education and Supervision, 1969, 8, 265-272 (c).

Carkhuff, R.R. & Berenson, B.G. Beyond counseling and
     therapy. New York: Holt, Rinehart, and Winston,
     1967.

Combs, A.W. A perceptual view of the adequate personality.
     In A.W. Combs (Ed.) Perceiving, behaving, becoming:
     Yearbook of the Association for supervison and
     curriculum development, 1962.

Dick, L.D. & Ragland, R.E. A study of meditation in the
     service of counseling. Unpublished manuscript,
     University of Oklahoma, 1973.

Drennen, W.T. & Chermol, B.H. Relaxation and placebo-
     suggestion as uncontrolled variables in TM research.
     Journal of Humanistic Psychology, (in press).

Eysenck, H.J. The effects of psychotherapy: An evaluation.
     Journal of Consulting Psychology, 1952, 16, 319-324.

Eysenck, H.J. The effects of psychotherapy. In H.J. Eysenck (Ed.) Handbook of Abnormal Psychology, New York: Basic Books, 1961.

Foulds, M.L. An investigation of the relationship between therapeutic conditions offered and a measure of self-actualization. Doctoral dissertation, University of Florida, 1967.

French, A.P. & Tupin, J.P. Method of relaxation. Journal of the American Medical Association, 1973, 223, 801-802.

French, A.P. & Tupin, J.P. Therapeutic application of a simple relaxation method. American Journal of Psychotherapy, 1974, 28, 282-287.

Goleman, D. Meditation as meta-therapy: Hypothesis toward a proposed fifth state of consciousness. Journal of Transpersonal Psychology, 1971, 3, 1-25.

Goleman, D. Meditation as meta-therapy. In J. White (Ed.) What is meditation? Garden City, N.J.: Doubleday, 1974.

Hjelle, L.A. Transcendental Meditation and psychological health. Perceptual and Motor Skills, 1974, 39, 623-628.

Holder, T. Length of Encounter as a therapist variable. Journal of Clinical Psychology, 1968, 24, 249-250.

Ilardi, R.I. & May, W.T. A reliability study of Shostrom's Personal Orientation Inventory. Journal of Humanistic Psychology, 1968, 68-72.

Kagan, N. & Krathwohl, D.R. Studies in human interaction: Interpersonal process recall stimulated by video tape. East Lansing, Michigan: Educational Publication Services, Michigan State University, 1967.

Kanellakos, D.P. & Ferguson, P.C. The psychobiology of transcendental meditation (An annotated bibliography). Los Angeles: MIU Press, 1973.

Kanellakos, D.P. & Lukas, J.S. The psychobiology of transcendental meditation: A literature review. Menlo Park, Ca.: W.A. Benjamin, 1974.

Keefe, T. Empathy: Impact of social work education and enhancement technique. Doctoral dissertation, University of Utah, 1973.

Knapp, R.R. Relationship of a measure of self-actualization
        to neuroticism and extraversion. Journal of Consulting
        Psychology, 1965, 29, 168-172.

Lesh, T.V. Zen meditation and the development of empathy
        in counselors. Journal of Humanistic Psychology, 1970,
        10, 39-74.

Luborsky, L., Auerback, A.H., Chandler, M., Cohen, H. &
        Backrach, J.M. Factors influencing the outcome of
        psychotherapy: A review of quantitative research.
        Psychological Bulletin, 1971, 75, 145-185.

Maslow, A.H. Motivation and Personality. New York: Harper,
        1954.

Maslow, A.H. Toward a psychology of being. Princeton: Van
        Nostrand, 1962.

McPheeters, H.L. & King, J.B. Plans for teaching mental
        health workers community college curriculum objectives.
        Atlanta: Southern Regional Education Board, 1971.

Morgan, J.I. Introduction to Paraprofessional training:
        Function, methods and issues. In J.I. Morgan (Ed.)
        Psychological and Vocational Counseling Center Mono-
        graph Series Vol. 2. Psychological and Vocational
        Counseling Center and Division of Continuing Education.
        University of Florida, Gainesville, 1976.

Naranjo, C. Meditation: Its spirit and technique. In
        Naranjo & R.E. Ornstein, On the psychology of medita-
        tion. New York: Viking, 1971.

Nidich, S., Seeman, W. & Dreskin, F. Influence of tran-
        scendental meditation: A replication. Journal of
        Counseling Psychology, 1973, 20, 565-566.

Piaget, G.W., Berenson, G.W. & Carkhuff, R.R. Differential
        effects of the manipulation of therapeutic conditions
        by high- and moderate-functioning therapists upon high
        and low functioning clients. Journal of Consulting
        Psychology, 1967, 31, 481-486.

Rogers, C.R. The necessary and sufficient conditions of
        therapeutic personality change. Journal of Consulting
        Psychology, 1957, 21, 95-103.

Rogers, C.R. On becoming a person. Boston: Houghton
        Miffling, 1961.

Russie, R.E. The influence of transcendental meditation
    on positive mental health and self-actualization and
    the role of expectation, rigidity and self-control in
    the achievement of these benefits. Doctor disserta-
    tion, California School of Professional Psychology,
    1975.

Schauble, P., Pierce, R. & Resnikoff, A. Measurement of
    counselor effectiveness. Comparison of dichotomous
    and continuous rating scales. Unpublished manuscript,
    1976.

Seeman, W., Nidich, S. & Banta, T. Influence of transcen-
    dental meditation on a measure of self-actualization.
    Journal of Counseling Psychology, 1972, 19, 184-187.

Shaffii, M. Adaptive and therapeutic aspects of meditation.
    International Journal of Psychoanalytic Psychotherapy,
    1973, 2, 364-382.

Shostrom, E.L. A test for the measurement of self-
    actualization. Educational and Psychological Measure-
    ment, 1964, 24, 207-218.

Shostrom, E.L. Manual for the Personal Orientation Inventory.
    San Diego, Calif.: Educational and Industrial Testing
    Service, 1966.

Shostrom, E.L. & Knapp, R.R. The relationship of a measure
    of self-actualization (POI) to a measure of pathology
    (MMPI) and to therapeutic growth. American Journal of
    Psychotherapy, 1966, 20, 193-202.

Siegel, S. Nonparametric statistics for the behavioral
    sciences. McGraw Hill Book Co., Inc., N.Y., 1956.

Thigpen, J.D. Most and least helpful experiences in the
    supervision of paraprofessional mental health workers.
    Doctoral dissertation, University of Florida, 1974.

Truax, C.B. The process of group psychotherapy: Relation-
    ship between hypothesized therapeutic conditions and
    intrapersonal exploration. Psychological Monogram,
    1961, 75, 7 (Whole No 511) (a).

Truax, C.B. A scale for the measurement of accurate empathy.
    Psychiatric Institute Bulletin, Wisconsin Psychiatric
    Institute, University of Wisconsin, 1961, I, issue 12
    (b).

Truax, C.B. A tentative scale for the measurement of therapist genuineness or self-congruence. Discussion Papers, Wisconsin Psychiatric Institute, University of Wisconsin, 1962, No 35 (a).

Truax, C.B. A tentative scale for the measurement of unconditional positive regard. Psychiatric Institute Bulletin, Wisconsin Psychiatric Institute, University of Wisconsin, 1962, No 2, issue No 1 (b).

Truax, C.B. & Carkhuff, R.R. Toward effective counseling and practice. Chicago, Ill., Aldine, 1967.

Truax, C.B., Silber, L. & Wargo, D. Personality change and achievement in therapeutic training. Unpublished manuscript, Arkansas Rehabilitation Research and Training Center, University of Arkansas, 1966.

Truax, C.B. & Tatum, C. An extension from the effective psychotherapeutic model to constructive personality change in preschool children. Childhood Education, 1966, 42, 456-462.

Wallace, R.K. Physiological effects of transcendental meditation. Science, 1970, 167, 1751-1754 (a).

Wallace, R.K. The physiological effects of transcendental meditation. A proposed fourth state of consciousness. Los Angeles: MIU Press, 1970 (b).

Wallace, R.K., Benson, H. & Wilson, A.F. A wakeful hypometabolic state. American Journal of Physiology, 1971, 221, 795-799.

Wehr, M. A study of the relationship between group facilitative involvement and predicted effectiveness of counselor paraprofessionals. Doctoral dissertation, University of Florida, 1973.

BIOGRAPHICAL SKETCH

David Nelson Bole was born July 26, 1949, in Detroit, Michigan. He attended a Catholic elementary school until his family moved to settle in Lake Worth, Florida. There he completed his public school education and was graduated from Lake Worth Senior High School in 1967. Later that same year he attended Palm Beach Junior College in Lake Worth, Florida, where he received his A.A. degree in 1969. In September of 1969 David attended the University of Florida in Gainesville, Florida, where he received his B.A. degree in psychology in 1971. He continued his education at the University of Florida in the Foundations of Education. After receiving his M.Ed. in June, 1972, he was accepted in the Ph.D. program in the Foundations of Education Department emphasizing Human Growth and Development. In August of 1974 he joined the faculty as a full-time psychology instructor in the Human Service Department at Greenville Technical College. Here he taught psychology, counseling, and directed Student Field Placements. He developed and led inservice teacher training programs for the Greenville Co. School System in communication skills and in behavior management. After remaining in this teaching position for two years, David left Greenville to finish his doctoral studies program at the University of Florida.

David specializes in the area of personal growth, bringing together the Eastern and Western theories of personality through an experiential orientation to education. David has studied Eastern psychologies, yoga, Tai Chi Chuan, relaxation methods, body awareness, and health in the United States, Canada, and India. He is also a licensed massage therapist and offers workshops designed to enhance awareness and health.

I certify that I have read this study and that in my opinion it conforms to acceptable standards of scholarly presentation and is fully adequate, in scope and quality, as a dissertation for the degree of Doctor of Philosophy.

Donald L. Avila, Chairman
Professor
Foundations of Education

I certify that I have read this study and that in my opinion it conforms to acceptable standards of scholarly presentation and is fully adequate, in scope and quality, as a dissertation for the degree of Doctor of Philosophy.

Walter Busby
Assistant Professor
Foundations of Education

I certify that I have read this study and that in my ipinion it conforms to acceptable standards of scholarly presentation and is fully adequate, in scope and quality, as a dissertation for the degree of Doctor of Philosophy.

Richard Anderson
Professor of Psychology

This dissertation was submitted to the Graduate Faculty of the Department of Foundations of Education in the College of Education and to the Graduate Council, and was accepted as partial fulfillment of the requirements for the degree of Doctor of Philosophy.

March 1978

Chairman, Foundations of Education

Dean, Graduate School